The

Immortality Guide

(200 Revolutionary Health Insites for Eternal Health and Long Life)!

By Dr.Moo-Twahz

The Peoples Healer Health Ministries

www.thepeopleshealer.com

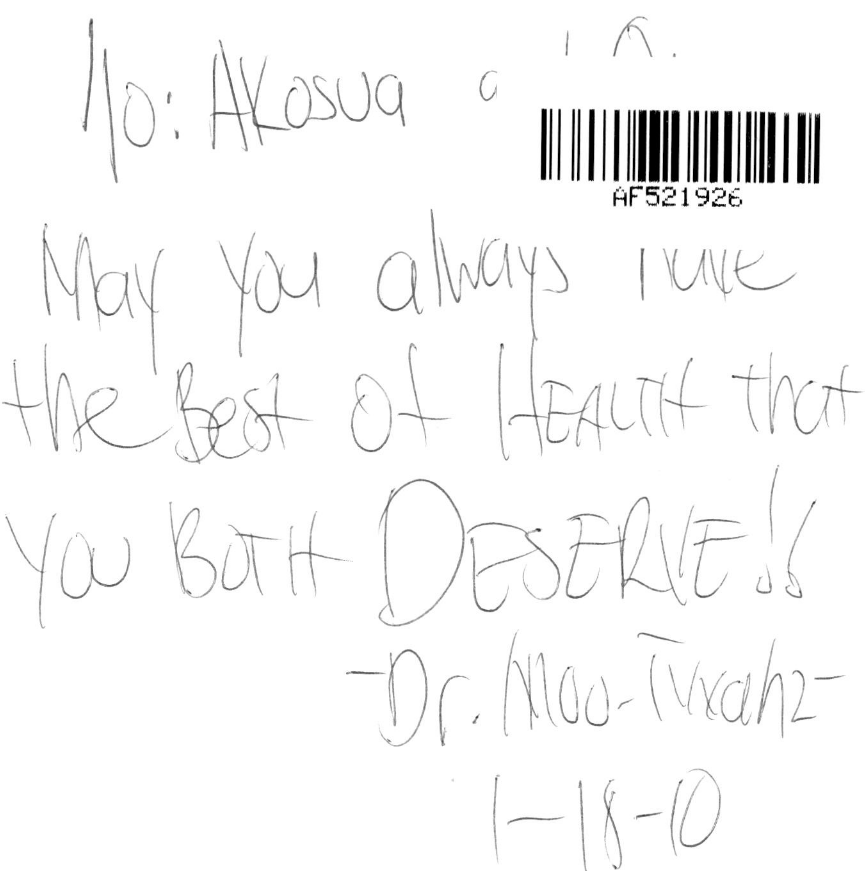

Published by TPH Media, P O Box 1883, St. Louis, MO 63118

Cover Design by SONN somethinofnothin.net

Photo by Herakhuty

DEDICATION

This book is DEDICATED to my BABA (RIP), the MAN who first brought me into Consciousness and who taught me everything I know about HEALING; My MAMA who was the first to open my mind to the written word; My CHILDREN: AKEEBULAN (The Thinking One), YIFTA (The Intellectual One), NAFTALI (The Magical One), ONDIECKHIR (The Fashionable One) and TECLA (The Visual One); By Babies Mama OLIVIA (aka MS. PAIN the FUNNIEST woman NOT doing Comedy and the first REAL friend I ever had who believed in me when no one else did), My Big Brotha DR. SUNSTAR (aka the Metaphysical Master of Mental Healing), My WIFE/RIGHT HAND WOMAN/AGENT/MANAGER, the one and only HERAKHUTY (aka MISTRESS NIGRESS)who has kept my MESSAGE from being buried and is the MAIN reason you are reading this work right now); and to ALL OF YOU who have SUPPORTED my HEALTH MINISTRY and INSPIRED me to do GREAT WORK for THE PEOPLE. Im GRATEFUL for all of YOU!

Dr. Moo-Twahz

The

Immortality Guide

(200 Revolutionary Healthy Insites for Eternal Health & Long Life)!

By Dr.Moo-Twahz

Founder, The Peoples Healer Health Ministries

www.thepeopleshealer.com

PREFACE

Our ANCESTERS looked to Natural HEALERS living among them to Heal Mind, Body, Soul and Spirit. These DEDICATED INDIVIDUALS helped people because it was their CALLING to do so. We live in a very different world today and the CONNECTION between the past and the present has been lost. However, the work of DR. MOO-TWAHZ bridges this gap.

DR. MOO-TWAHZ, descending from a long line of FOLK HEALERS and ROOT WORKERS, is a self-taught 6th Generation HEALER and Spiritual Advisor with ANCIENT SOULutions for the MODERN WORLD. He draws upon ANCESTRAL KNOWLEDGE to help people heal themselves naturally. This commitment to helping people from all walks of life - of all ethnicities, creeds or religion - has earned him the title: *The PEOPLES HEALER.*

Dr. Moo-Twahz is an OUTSPOKEN, PLAIN TALKING, FUNNY, CONTROVERSIAL, CHARISMATIC TEACHER of NATURAL HEALING and SPIRITUALITY. His RADICAL views on modern day MEDISIN; UNUSUAL work using simple FRUITS and FOODS for HEALING; and unorthodox SPIRITUAL philosophy–have been RESTORING people back to HEALTH everywhere he goes!

Dr. MOO-TWAHZ speaks/lectures all over the world. Originally from Southern Tennessee, he now lives in Saint Louis, MO.

The IMMORTALITY GUIDE

(200 Revolutionary Health Insights for Eternal Health & Long Life)!
By Dr. Moo-Twahz

"It would appear as if man is really UNABLE to SUSTAIN life without either MEAT or MILK and MILK PRODUCTS. Anyone who DECEIVES people in this regard or countenances is a FRAUD and an ENEMY of INDIA."
--MAHATMA GHANDI--
(commenting on the Dangers of the Vegan lifestyle)

"The Body is a HUMAN PLANT. And as such we need the same nourishment: SUNLITE, WATER, OXYGEN and good SOIL (Gut Flora) to flourish."
--Dr. Moo-Twahz—

INTRODUCTION

This book is because we must Teach OUR SELFS How To EAT all Over Again. We must Teach our selfs how to HEAL all over again. The MEDICAL establishment, the HOSPITAL INDUSTRIAL COMPLEX, the PHARMAKOS/DRUG DEALERS of WALLSTREET, the New World Order OLIGARCHIES, the HIPPIE HEALTH COMMUNE, the RAW FOODISTS, the VEGANS and VEGETARIANS have all filled our heads with HALF-TRUTHS and LIES (knowingly or UNKNOWINGLY) in order that we may worship at their DRUG TEMPLES and/or their GREED-DRIVEN, LAW OF ATTRACTION HEALTHFOOD STORES. They have CONSTIPATED our minds with REGURGITATED Shit Lit from so-called Natural Health AUTHORS/DOKTORS whose IDEAS were RONG or MISGUIDED to begin with!

It is Time to CHANGE! However, let me WARN You--it WILL NOT make you POPULAR (just like it has not made ME popular— or WELCOME in certain so-called HEALTH CIRCLES). This information has come thru me to you. Yet, Im only a CONDUIT—YOU must DO IT! If the change is to be effective-- Only you can save YOU from those who would rob YOU of your birthrite to ETERNAL HEALTH and LONG LIFE by trying to STARVE you to Death with Totally GRASS-FED Diets (apparently, they see you as a COW); or KILL you in their HORSEpitals with ARSENIC-based MEDS! Rather than advise a well-rounded, LIVE, WHOLE FOODS Eating Regimen that includes Nutrition from MORE of the FOOD groups. This is a fight for the HEALTH and LONGEVITY of your BODY, MIND, SPIRIT and SOUL. One you Must WIN!

--Dr. Moo-Twahz—
January 2010

FOREWORD

YOU are no longer in an age of SLOW ADAPTATION (time is coming) rather one of FAST MUTATION (time is here). You no longer have the luxury of waiting for Adaptation. You must embrace Mutation. Rather than wait on CHANGE--You must BE THE CHANGE you do NOT see! Failure to Adapt has always caused a SPECIES to become EXTINCT (Dinosaurs). And so it is with HUMANITY as well. And so it is with YOU! Seek you therefore to Pull into your BODY all the FOODS and THOUGHTS of the HIGHEST VIBRATION that are in ALIGNMENT with those of the Increasing FREQUENCY of MAMA EARTH. This means your EATING and THINKING will have to be of the highest REVOLUTIONARY order it can be. Just like the INSITES in this book, it is time to go to the next phase in this New World Order. *What we call DISEASE is really a SYMPTOM. One that is LOCKED UP in our CELLS. And the SOULUTION is to OPEN that cell with the Rite SKELETON KEY (Nutrient) and RELEASE the Disease so that it will go back from whence it came. Then you will heal.* Keep this book by your bedside so you can refer to it often as you seek to MOTIVATE your Body through the HEALING process.

REVOLUTIONARY HEALTH INSITE #0: **The HUMAN BODY has Evolved to Eat MEAT! And has been Evolved to do so for quite a long time. According to FOSSIL FOOD RECORDS, Humanity EVOLVED the ability to eat Meat about 2 million years ago (after that FALL FROM GRACE which happened at some unknown date in the distant past) In other words, there has NEVER been a time in the most recent past that we have NOT eaten MEAT!** One would have to go back past that 2 million years ago to find a time when EVOLUTION did not favor us eating MEAT; rather we were more SUSTAINED off the RAYS of the SUN.

The PROBLEM with our Meat-Eating selves today, however, is that we eat TOO MUCH meat! You see, it is the OVERCONSUMPTION and lack of QUALITY of the MEAT(not the EATING of Meat itself) which forces our bodies to use up TOO much NITROGEN and produces Excessive URIC ACID! Most of us are eating twice our WEIGHT in Meat per year! (You only need approximately 25% of your weight in meat per year to thrive).

Yet at the MUCH smaller, RATIONAL amount--we actually BENEFIT from URIC ACID in Meat which is one of the most little-known, yet POWERFUL ANTIOXIDANTS in our food arsenal (*CARNOSINE* being another)! Meat, however, is best served via BOILING/STEWING/SLOW COOKING in order for the BODY to utilize it most effectively. BOILING/STEWING/SLOW COOKING actually SEALS in the Juices and NUTRIENTS. (Frying and BBQing makes meat poisonous).

The idea that we all must be VEGANS is a feeding strategy that is ILLING and/or KILLING people of all ETHNICITIES! The ALL-PLANT, RAW FOODS/VEGAN Diet is ESPECIALLY "not" for the

BLACK MAN & WOMAN! In general, Black people are definitely one group of Ethnic people who, absolutely, positively NEED, at least SOME MEAT!! A little Meat. Not that much. But we DO need it. A VEGAN DIET for life will TAKE the Average Black persons life!! There are CO-FACTORS in Meat such as CARNOSINE and URIC ACID (which has been sold as being BAD, however, is in fact, a Supreme ANTIOXIDANT of the first order. And you will find its presence in LONG LIVED people the world over)! And you can not and will not FIND these vital nutrients in PLANT FOODS.

Letz deal with our WHITE BRETHEREN/SISTREN for a minute. As a Rule WHITE people are more suited to VEGAN Diets due to their A & AB BloodTypes----AND----their GEOGRAPHICAL HERITAGE (COLD CLIMATE where you will find a higher CODING for A Bloodtypes which can survive mo better off GRASS! Whereas most BLACK people are linked GEOGRAPHICALLY to a HOT CLIMATE and an O Bloodtype—meaning survival needs to include MEAT)! *Yes, some Black people can cross over to VEGANISM due to having Bloodtype A,* however, the BLOOD is not the ONLY factor. Again, we have to factor in GEOGRAPHICAL LINEAGE, METABOLISM, ANCESTRY—and our old favorite: MELANIN—all which Influences the FOODS that can best be eaten by YOU in particular and by an individual ETHNIC GROUP in general.

It must be understood that every Ethnic Group has evolved a STOMACH FLORA that is more suited to what they MUST eat to be Healthy. This is a GENETIC ADAPTION that carries over via BLOOD, ANCESTRY, LOCATION and ENVIRONMENT (EPIGENETICS/NUTRIGENOMICS). In short, if ANYBODY is MEANT to be a TOTAL PLANT-eating, RAW FOOD, VEGAN—it is a WHITE MAN or WOMAN. Based on GUT FLORA, BLOODTYPE and GEOGRAPHICAL ANCESTRY: this is more the WHITE

PROFILE. So BLACK PEOPLE please quit letting WHITE PEOPLE Tell yawl how to EAT TO LIVE on GRASS and GRAVEL (grains)!

The many HEALTH problems that Black people have can be traced to eating out of their ETHNIC and GEOGRAPHICAL Heritage! A Vegan Diet (which can be useful for cleaning on a short-term basis) is essentially a STARVATION DIET! Something to subsist off of until you can get some MEAT! A lone individual (or few individuals) may be able to SURVIVE off eating ONLY plant foods, grains, nuts, seeds and berries. However, there is no way, you will be able to KEEP an entire CIVILIZATION of people alive (and HEALTHY with a LONG LIFESPAN) with just those foods. MEAT has to figure into the picture somewhere. And SOONER rather than Later! And here is the kicker: you do NOT need that MUCH meat to accomplish this! However, you DO. NEED. MEAT!

Any CIVILIZATION/CULTURE of PEOPLE of at least the last 20,000 years that has tried to SURVIVE with NO MEAT at all (by attempting VEGANISM)—has not SURVIVED. *(If so, where are these VEGAN CIVILIZATIONS)?* NO BABIES can be born without the INTRINSIC FACTORS of Meat. NO HORMONES can be made without the FAT of MEAT. Thus, NO FERTILITY (this is what <and is> one of the problems of WHITE WOMEN and their INFERTILITY problems—even to this day--NO FAT). Historically, WHITE PEOPLE died off and had shorter lifespans because they could not find ANIMALS to eat in their Cold, Harsh CLIMATE. Therefore, NO CHILDREN. And INFERTILE women----and MEN. This EVOLVED more of an A and AB BLOODTYPE among them(and WHITE BLOOD CELLS….whereas Black People have Less WHITE BLOOD CELLS in general). In other words, a STARVATION DIET based on ROOTS, PLANTS, SHRUBS, WEEDS, NUTS, SEEDS (whenever the weather changed some or relented to allow something to grow). The EVOLUTIONARY affect on the White Persons GUT FLORA is a type of STOMACH ACID that can squeeze out more NUTRIENTS from PLANT FOODS than can the Stomach of a BLACK PERSON! Not only that, Less SUN was available which also influenced not only BONE DENSITY, but BLOODTYPE ---- AND ----FERTILITY. Caint have children without the SUN!!

This is why its CRUCIAL to overstand your PERSONAL history and connection to your ETHNICITY! You may be trying to be a VEGAN when its simply impossible for you to be ONE! And you are ILLing and KILLing yourself and ENDANGERING your CHILDREN as well!!

So what am I saying? Im saying you can do just as well on a EATIQUETTE (diet) of 60%-80% VEGETABLES, FRUITS, SEEDS and NUTS—as long as the last 20%-40% includes a small ration of MEAT and MEAT BY-PRODUCTS (RAW CHEESE, EGGS, BUTTER and RAW MILK when you can get it directly). On an eating Regimen of such—the LONGEST LIVED PEOPLE in the world are testament to this day of such FOODS! And such a RATIO. This is one similarity ALL long-lived ethnicities have ACROSS THE BOARD (regardless of RACE): they eat SMALL portions of Meat. However, they eat the FOODS of *their* ANCESTORS! You would do well to at least investigate such a longevity eating plan.

Furthermore, your ETHNICITY (ANCESTRY) is the PRIMARY means that determines your EATIQUETTE (diet) and how you should be HEALED whenever you fall sick! The following EPIGENETIC OVERRIDES "must" be FACTORED in as well: BLOODTYPE, GENDER TYPE, METABOLIC TYPE, ENVIRONMENT, GEOGRAPHICAL/CLIMATE HERITAGE. Thus, you may be BLACK but have a LINK to ASIAN, INDIAN and yes, WHITE heritages. And this will AFFECT what you "must" EAT and how you "must" TREAT (heal) your BODY. For example, in general, the Best OIL for a BLACK PERSON is COCONUT OIL or BUTTER OIL; for a WHITE PERSON—CODLIVER OIL or BUTTER OIL; for a

AMERINDIAN PERSON—SESAME OIL; and for a LATIN PERSON—OLIVE OIL. Your DIET should NOT be based on what the WORLD or SOCIETY is doing. Rather it should be based on the aforementioned AREAS—because this will give YOU a CLUE what works best for YOU. And not what everybody else is EATING! For most of us, especially, *BLACK PEOPLE, a VEGAN DIET is a STARVATION DIET!* So stay away from being a TOTAL Vegan until you investigate thoroughly whether or not its truly for you. Otherwise, you can make yourself truly SICK! And your children if you have them! Continue to include a little MEAT in your eating habits WHILE you are investigating how long you want to eat as a Total VEGAN if ever (which can have tremendous benefits as a form of ACTIVE Healing, yet, not as a long term form of eating for most of us)! (see Insite #40, 45, 49).

REVOLUTIONARY HEALTH INSITE #1: **Most important LIVE, WHOLE FOOD NUTRIENTS currently in the world today are IODINE (infection/thyroid), SELENIUM (immunity/thymus), IRON (blood creation), BORON (bone marrow), VITAMIN D (bone density), VITAMIN K (blood glue), LECITHIN (brain food), CHOLESTEROL (prevents alzheimers/protects cells), SEROTONIN (mood), SULFUR (pancreas strength), STRONTIUM (bones...the strongest bones contain adequate Strontium), CESIUM (cell life/respiration), VANADIUM (pancreas, keeps protein in muscles, myoglobin)!** The societal environment of the modern world is not Beneficial enough to the HUMAN PLANT. And with the coming EARTH CHANGES (movement thru PHOTON BELT, GLOBAL WARMING)—the ORGAN requirements for ALL Minerals have become extremely CRITICAL for well-being!

REVOLUTIONARY HEALTH INSITE #2: **DRINK COLD (distilled) WATER to Stop SUGAR CRAVINGS.** The COLDNESS of the DISTILLED Water cools out the HYPOTHALAMUS GLAND (which controls APPETITE and CRAVINGS) for 10-20 seconds at a time, shutting down the CRAVING. 1-2 times when the CRAVE hits you should be sufficient. (see Insite# 26)

REVOLUTIONARY HEALTH INSITE #3: **GAZE AT THE MOON TO HEAL ANEMIA.**

Gazing at the MOON, especially, a FULL MOON, during the hours of 11pm-2am, will increase the IRON stores in your BLOOD. The effects that can be gained from MOON GAZING are just as BENEFICIAL as SUN GAZING. Do both of them. Short periods, of time (blinking at the Sun); longer periods of time staring at the MOON. Best to find a HIGH, CLEAR place (Hill, Mountain, Cliff, Rooftop) and stare UN-INTERRUPTED for long as you can. The Moon has MAGNETISM which reacts with the SOFT Iron in your Blood—producing more of the same. The nighttime moon creates IONS in the ATMOSPHERE that act on the BLOOD (and thus Body proper) to create balance. 10pm-2am is the most optimum time period.

REVOLUTIONARY HEALTH INSITE #4: **GAZE AT THE SUN TO HEAL AIDS.**

Gazing at the SUN: NEW (morning)....RIPE (evening) SUN during the hours of RISING and SETTING Sun—as well as the HIGH NOON Sun, will produce more of an ACTIVE form of VITAMIN D (D-3, which KILLS off AUTO-IMMUNE INFECTIONS). SUN BATHING at HIGH NOON for very, short periods of 10-12 minutes is also a KRUCIAL CURE-AID. Use VIRGIN COCONUT OIL (BLACK PEOPLE), SESAME SEED OIL (AMERINDIANS, INDIANS, ASIANS); EXTRA VIRGIN OLIVE OIL (LATINOS/HISPANICS); or CODLIVER OIL (WHITE PEOPLE). HIV/AIDS along with HEPATITIS, TUBERCULOSIS and many other so-called AUTO-IMMUNE dis-eases--all have a connection with ACTIVATED VITAMIN D DEFICIENCY. Obtaining a UVB LIGHT is also good (or tanning for very short periods) for Vite D synthesis.

REVOLUTIONARY HEALTH INSITE #5: **OIL/FAT (especially SATURATED FAT) SLOWS AGING and is the best FUEL for the Body. We have been sold/told that the best fuel is CARBOHYDRATE SUGAR which is a blatant LIE or just pure IGNORANCE)!** Especially, REFINED CARBS are DANGEROUS! *(see also Insite #6)* A simple tablespoon of SATURATED OIL (like BUTTER or COCONUT OIL) strengthens your BLOOD CELL MEMBRANE (outer and inner covering). This PROTECTS it from CELLULAR fallout aka FREE RADICALS that happen when other cells around it explode when they BURN out. Like avoiding SHRAPNEL from a BOMB. The FALLOUT just bounces off of the Protected CELL. The OIL also keeps the CELL from AGING due to it being FLEXIBLE, PERMEABLE and therefore has the ability to STRETCH and accommodate BODILY CHANGES. This allows it to LAST LONGER. Which means YOU last longer and AGE SLOWER. Additionally, OIL causes your body to CREATE more CELLS when under stress (meaning while FREE RADICALS are causing FALL OUT, the OIL is causing BUILD UP of new cells at a ratio of 6:1 *(my stats),* for every 1 cell that is DESTROYED by FREE RADICALS, Oil creates 6 newer ones). Again, this SLOWS Aging. The length of time your cells are able to REPLICATE(its HAYFLICK LIMIT) before Dying (APOPTOSIS) increases significantly. Work your way up to DRINKING at least 4 ounces of Oil per week. INORGANIC (from Fried, Heated oils) SUFFOCATES the BLOOD CELL which is why FAT can often be found in CANCER CELLS! Organic FAT/OIL on the other hand TRANSMITS RESONANCE to the CELL allowing for longer CELL LIFE! A True DURA(able)CELL!!

Of course, You want to watch out for the KILLER FATS known as TRANSFATS which are a PLAGUE on the Health of the PEOPLE! In fact, it is a downrite KILLER of people. Yet, the FDA let this KHEMICAL be invented so that people could Eat! (Follow the money....the FDA is an organization that lets a company submit their own research that validates their product; meanwhile the FDA never even double checks the research).

Is nobody in their rite minds studying what this POISON does to the CELLS of HUMANS? Its NOT even a real FAT/OIL--it may MIMIC fat. Yet, its not a FAT at all. Its a PLASTIK FORMALDEHYDE! This stuff was made to KILL off your BLOOD CELLS on purpose--or else we have some really DUMB scientists who dont know what the hell they are doing in the laboratory (its one or the other)!

Letz look at the backstory to OILS/FAT:
FATS are either SATURATED or UNSATURATED. Saturated meaning lots of HYDROGEN spread across its khemical bonds; UNSATURATED meaning LITTLE or NO HYDROGEN spread across its khemical bonds. The more HYDROGEN--the better because HYDROGEN is (a) the SOURCE of LIFE (ala the SUN which is nothing but a big ball of Hydrogen....so u can see this Hydrogen is important)! Conversely, the LESS hydrogen--the WORSE. In other words, the MORE Saturated a Fat is--the better it is for your body due to the amount of HYDROGEN it contains (its like EATING THE SUN)!!
(SIDENOTE: this should tell you then that SATURATED FATS which come mostly from ANIMAL FOODS are the best FATS! (including BUTTER). Some FRUITS have these FATS or close to these Fats, and I recommend them, ie., COCONUTS, AVOCADOES, OLIVES, SEEDS).

Back to FAT ANALYSIS.

The QUALITY and the HEALTHINESS of the Fat for the Human Body also depends whether or not the FAT/OIL has a KINK in it. SMALL KINK or NO KINK is what you want because this means the OIL can be ABSORBED into the CELL much easier. And this builds CELL INTEGRITY, the MEMBRANE, helps the CELL REGENERATE. Once again, this honor goes mostly to SATURATED ANIMAL FATS! and to a lesser degree MONOUNSATURATED PLANT FATS (Olive Oil, for example, which is indeed good oil, however, its NOT as SATURATED as ANIMAL and/or BUTTER FAT--and thus has LESS HYDROGEN). The ability of SATURATED FAT to get directly into the cell EXTENDS Cell lifespan, helping it to have more REPLICATIONS or TURNOVERS before it DIES (aka APOPTOSIS); and protects it during OXIDATION from FREE RADICALS.

Well, here is the EVILNESS of TRANSFAT created by these FRANKENMEDS!---- It has NO KINKS, either yawl!!!!. REPEATING: NO----DAMN----KINKS!!!! Thus it FOOLS your CELLS into believing it is a REAL fat! And not only that but a GOOD FAT (good lawd that is just plain RONG); and so the CELL allows it to COME INSIDE. However, once inside it DESTROYS the LIQUID (cytoplasm) inside the cell!! This is the type of FAT that MOLECULAR BIOLOGISTS are finding in CANCER CELLS now! Its TRANSFAT (and/or HEATED FAT/OIL). Which has exploded the Cell, leaving its FRAGMENTED GENETIC fingerprint all over it! This is the same action of any KILLER VIRUS as well! It copies the GENOME of a REGULAR cell----yet is NOT a Regular Cell---its a MUTANT CELL....DO NOT EAT THIS SHIZZ----EVER!!!!

ADDENDUM: Dont believe the Hype AGAINST Saturated Fats (meaning, of course from, GRASS-FED, ORGANIC clean MEATS). Your Cells are MOSTLY Saturated Fat. And so are your ORGANS. Especially, the LIVER and the HEART (in fact, this is why CODLIVER OIL is recommend to recovering HEART ATTACK patients--to rebuild that SATURATED FAT around it--and to increase the viability of NITROGEN SYNTHESIS that YOUR heart desperately needs to function properly).

If YOU include LIVE, WHOLE, ORGANIC FOODS from all Food Sources, ie., MEAT, FRUITS, VEGETABLES, SEEDS, WATER, EGGS, MILK--you INCREASE your chances of obtaining all the proper, VARIED amounts of FATS that your CELLS need. Especially SATURATED FAT.

The body EVOLVED to run off Fat *(creating a state of KETOSIS).* Yet, we have destroyed this MECHANISM OF ACTION on a CARBO DIET, leading to a SUGAR ADDICTION. Meanwhile, still convinced by the GATE KEEPERS of Health that GLUCOSE via CARBS is the main fuel for our BRAINS! Not true. It is via FAT. Yes! NOT Carbohydrates. (which is what we get not only from refined CARBS; but in all VEGAN/RAW FOOD Diets which just amounts to STARCH and SURGAR). (See Insite #6)

REVOLUTIONARY HEALTH INSITE #6: **CARBOHYDRATES (especially, REFINED ones) are the worst source of ENERGY/FUEL for the body in comparison to FATS (and they are just as much of a KILLER of the Entire HUMAN RACE as TRANSFATS and GRAINS)!!!!** *(*And DANGEROUS because due to GLUCOSE metabolism, they cause the CELLS of the Body to BURN UP quickly. This is AGING (a form of KETOACIDOSIS=something that kills DIABETICS usually from too much ACID in the BLOOD—and will KILL or IS killing you too from all those CARBS)!!

Yet, we have been told that we MUST consume CARBS to MAXIMIZE energy when this is in ERROR! Its just an attempt by CORPORATIONS and HOSPITALS to continue using you as a GUINEA PIG who PAYS them! The body simply can NOT use CARBS too often as a fuel because they OVERWORK the PANCREAS, forcing it to produce too much INSULIN and GLUCOSE which wears out your ORGANS.

CARBOHYDRATES take a lot of WATER to generate energy within the Body, ie., you need 4 tablespoons of WATER to 1 tablespoon of CARBS. Not so with FAT/OIL! (which actually GENERATES extra CELLS during METABOLISM). Thus, consuming Carbs MINIMIZES your energy and brings on SENILITY and OLD AGE at an extremely FAST rate! There is game being played with the BODIES of Humanity. They are offering us up to BUTCHERS (Doktors) feeding us on SUGAR which is slaying us at record rates. The body has Evolved to run off FAT *(creating a state of KETOSIS).* Yet, we have destroyed this MECHANISM on a CARBO DIET, leading to a SUGAR ADDICTION, still convinced by the GATE KEEPERS of Health that GLUCOSE via CARBS is the main fuel for our BRAINS! Not true.

Via FAT, yes. Not CARBOHYDRATES. Feed your BRAIN FAT that it breaks down into GLUCOSE which in turn helps it create MORE Neuronal connections—rather than SUGAR which KILLS off BRAIN CELLS (Alzheimers, Parkinsons)! (see Insites # 5, 18, 22, 45, 47, 200).

REVOLUTIONARY HEALTH INSITE #7: **COFFEE BOOSTS HUMAN GROWTH HORMONES.**

Just drinking 1-2 small cups of ORGANIC COFFEE per day promotes HORMONE GROWTH inclusive of ANDROGEN & TESTOSTERONE in men and ESTROGEN & PROGESTERONE in women. Add in nutrients like BERRIES or APPLE CIDER VINEGAR and you have one of the most POTENT ANTI-OXIDANTS ever! COFFEE also increases MELANIN STIMULATION, LIBIDO and VASCULAR strength. Use as a FACIAL to promote New SKIN growth for a YOUNGER look. This is the key thing: Do not make it a HABIT to drink COFFEE by itself too often (remember it is a MEDICINAL HERB)! However, mixed with BERRIES—it forms a very different phenomenal ELIXIR and ANTIOXIDANT that becomes LIFE GIVING rather than DRAINING the ADRENAL GLANDS! You can use it as an ENEMA to help clean the LIVER/GALL BLADDER and promote BILE (which then acts like, again an ANTIOXIDANT). Good-bye HEPATITIS!

REVOLUTIONARY HEALTH INSITE #8: **EXERCISE is Killing us more than it is Helping us extend our lives!** The reason why? We are EXHAUSTING our KIDNEYS, HEARTS and PANCREAS way too much! Every time you work out (much like when you eat) you TAX your ORGANS. They have to go into their RESERVES to PRESERVE you during that workout. On an occasional basis this is good. Like, say, every 4—6 days (even every 10 days is good, however be active doing something every day)! Then, it is great to REV up the body because this MIMICS ancient fight or flight mechanisms of the body which acted to give the body IMMUNITY via all the extra BLOOD and HORMONES produced. However, this was NOT something that was to happen constantly. Yet, this is exactly what we re-create when we WORK OUT everyday! And work out HARD too many times in a week. It is simply too MUCH. You FORCE the body to produce CORTISOL, ADRENALINE, GLUCOSE—all of which are STRESS DRUGS of the body. And their constant daily production results in the body being DESTROYED rather than BUILT UP!! Men/Women are LIFTING too heavy and running which forces a PROLAPSE (dropping) of the WOMB, OVARIES/TESTICLES and COLON (especially, the TRANSVERSE piping which goes across the abdomen). Also running is hard on the SPINE which can interfere with FERTILITY in both Women and Men (even ORGASM can be affected).

Note: I am NOT saying do not work out or exercise or avoid activity. Im saying keep it CASUAL! Get most of your exercise/activity being busy with LIFE (ie gardening). Walking around your city. Being ACTIVE. However, just you understand, in order for the BODY to LIVE LONG it does indeed have to be STRESSED (in MODERATION) and NOT that often! This is the KEY. Not this Constant WAR, wear and tear we put our bodies thru based on some workout program taught in basically every GYM/CENTER in the United States)! Are there people who are exceptions to this rule? Yes. Just like with eating. However, likewise, you must workout for your TYPE. In this case, the HUMAN TYPE does NOT need to work out everyday like s/he is going to WAR! It is okay to do so every now and then (like that 4-6 day schedule; even every 6-10 days mite be good for many of you). Keep it LOOSE and CASUAL. The hard driving-must -do workout ethic is why so many people feel they can't into shape. Its too much like a damn JOB! A workout should not be WORK! It should be fun. The name of the *LONGEVITY GAME is to REST more than WORK!*

The Following applies to MEN and WOMEN:
All WEIGHT LIFTING should be LIGHT (as a rule). If you want to RUN—do so only periodically. In fact, WALKING/RUNNING is best. Start off Walking. Then, Run a little bit. Back to walking and so on for only 20 minutes MINIMUM and 40 minutes MAXIMUM. This should only happen ONCE every 4-6 days! Always start off SMALL and work up to doing more. Be relaxed. Have fun. While you workout.

REVOLUTIONARY HEALTH INSITE #9: **HORMONES are how your Body Communicates with itself!** Your BLOOD CELLS are governed by HORMONIC DIALOGUE between the BRAIN and the OUTSIDE of the CELL (each Cell has ANTENNAE-like hairs on it that pick up FREQUENCIES in the form of SUBSTANCES secreted by the GLANDS in the Brain, i.e, FOLLICLE STIMULATING HORMONES or LUTEINIZING HORMONES for MENSTRUATION and BREASTFEEDING, for example). When all of this is working rite—your body is said to be in HORMONY (harmony). However, when your HORMONES are DISRUPTED by things like SUGAR and REFINED CARBOHYDRATES, BIRTH CONTROL PILLS, KHEMICALS, PRESERVATIVES, ADDITIVES, SMOKING, HORMONE REPLACEMENT THERAPY, BIO-IDENTICAL HORMONES (which are just more problems in the long run....better to put in the work to ADJUST your HORMONES naturally with FOOD rather than with those damn BIO-IDENTICAL HORMONE CREAMS)!! you can/will manifest a wide range of problems, usually, MENTAL/EMOTIONAL (everything from BIPOLARISM to DEPRESSION to MADNESS)—thus its key to have HORMONIC COOPERATION. If you just have to use BIO-IDENTICAL HORMONES you need to have an EATIQUETTE supported by hella good whole, live foods.
(see Insites # 6, 17).

REVOLUTIONARY HEALTH INSITE #10: **The BRAIN tends to BREAK DOWN on a Diet of GLUCOSE created by REFINED CARBOHYDRATES (processed flour, sugar, packaged goods, canned goods, and so on) rather than from FATS!** PSCIENCE tells us that this is the way the Brain MUST operate. Yet, this over-reliance on CARBS for Brain Fuel is destroying all of the NEURONAL CONNECTIONS in our HEADS due to the prevention of GLIAL CELLS (cells that help the formation of newer brain cells—thus producing Diseases such as MULTIPLE SCLEROSIS, ALZHEIMERS, PARKINSONS and MENTAL ILLNESS). Yes, the Brain needs GLUCOSE, however, it needs to be predominately created by the Breakdown of FATS in the form of KETONES (which is a SUGAR too that gets into the BRAIN) and has the EXACT same chemical reactions. Only its CLEANER and SAFER and does not DESTROY the Brain the way GLUCOSE from CARBS do! Thus, keep Carbs LOW, yet still NUTRIENT and PROTEIN-DENSE. And Fats HIGH *(Dr. ROBERT ATKINS was right all along....may he rest in PEACE).* In the final analysis, REFINED CARBS and HARD DRUGS create the same reaction, metabolically speaking, inside the body!! Thus, as far as your BODY is concerned—you are BURNING your brain out just as though you were SHOOTING UP the local STREET DRUG!

The KETONES are the main form of SUGAR that the body needs (created from FAT). It burns cleaner in the body proper and also activates the all-important GLUCAGON in the bloodstream! And this GLUCAGON is the flipside to the CORROSIVE EFFECT of GLUCOSE (and attendant INSULIN)! Furthermore, GLUCAGON switches on the PARASYMPATHETIC NERVOUS SYSTEM which allows the body to REST as it DIGESTS. Meanwhile, CARBS activate your body to use its STRESS-producing SYMPATHETIC

NERVOUS SYSTEM which does nothing but Wear Your Body Out as it creates overproduction of INSULIN and CORTISOL! (see Insite#5 & 6)

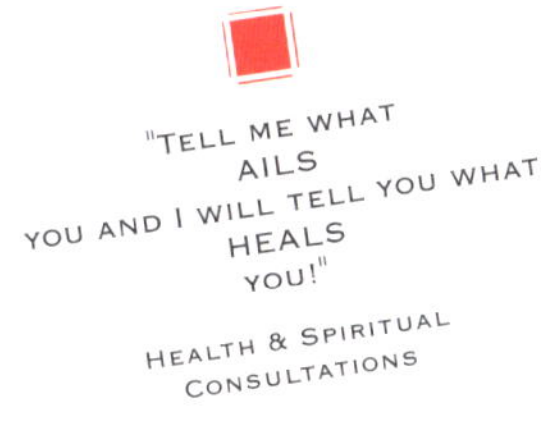

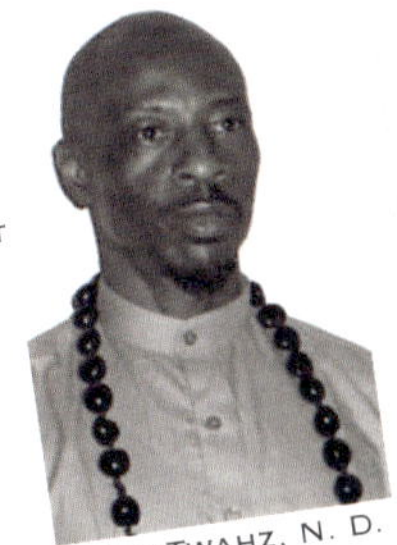

Fees Negotiable

Call Now: 314 802-8110
www.thepeopleshealer.com
www.youtube.com/mutwasze
www.blogtalkradio.com/manifestation

REVOLUTIONARY HEALTH INSITE #11: **BAKING SODA RAISES the PH/MOLECULAR VIBRATION of your WATER**. Thus, no need for ALKALINE, KANGEN, MICROPROCESSED or STRUCTURED waters all the health hypers are promoting, ceaselessly. All BOGUS marketing hype! For example, 1 gallon of distilled water will be BOOSTED by 1 level teaspoon of BAKING SODA (non-aluminum). This INCREASES the number of ELECTRONS in the water, which in turn gives it more OXYGEN and PROPER HOMEOSTATIC BALANCE (aka PH BALANCE). No need to buy KANGEN or some other specialized water. You can if you want. But this is a COST-EFFECTIVE way to do the same thing. Additionally, if you BOIL the water First then transfer it to GLASS JARS/STAINLESS STEEL containers after it kools—THEN putting in the BAKING SODA--you have BOOSTED its EFFECTIVENESS even more! Heat DISTILLS the water even further, making it more POTENT. Additional strategies, like putting your water in the sun boosts its potency.

REVOLUTIONARY HEALTH INSITE #12: **FERMENTED/SOUR FOODS increase BRAIN CELLS** because they increase BACTERIA in the DIGESTIVE SYSTEM which is connected to the NERVOUS SYSTEM housing the BRAIN (the BIGGEST single Nerve Cell in the body when you think about it)! The NUTRIENTS of Fermented/Sour Foods are taken up by both the DIGESTIVE TRACT and the NEURONS in the BRAIN. And this effects EMOTIONS and WELL-BEING. And letz not forget that these foods also confer IMMUNITY to the entire body. This is because the BACTERIA in the gut feed off of FERMENTED foods as means to their REPRODUCTION which in turn keeps you HEALTHY. These Healthy Bacteria secrete protective khemicals that act as barriers to any TOXINS in the system. (pointing to their effectiveness in healing health issues such as autism, multiple sclerosis). (see Insite #13).

REVOLUTIONARY HEALTH INSITE #13: **Drink only CERTIFIED, ORGANIC RAW COW/GOAT/SHEEP MILK (there are only a few approved places to get it from so that should not be a problem verifying its quality).** However, letz say you can only get PASTEURIZED MILK. Bring it home and POUR organic APPLE CIDER VINEGAR in it which will help RE-STERILIZE it and LIBERATE the remaining NUTRIENTS in it. And make it more DIGESTIBLE as a kinda FERMENTED/SOUR/BUTTERMILK (after you let it sit overnite). You are achieving the same thang as the idea behind YOGURT (with ACTIVE CULTURES). Of course, you can do the same thing with the RAW MILK and turn it into BUTTERMILK. (see Insite# 12)

REVOLUTIONARY HEALTH INSITE #14: **CHOLESTEROL should be on the HIGH side rather than the low side (upwards of 240 or more because the LONGEST LIVED <and allegedly the Most GENIUS> people have the Highest cholesterol)!** The Higher the CHOLESTEROL is in your body, the LONGER you will live. As you get OLDER, your Cholesterol amount goes up (to protect your VEINS which typically have started to DECAY from the onslaught of previous BAD eating......additionally, the more STRESS you are under the Higher your Cholesterol can be as well, even up over 300-plus....again, this is to PROTECT rather than WRECK you)! In general, you want to encourage HIGH cholesterol by eating Good SATURATED, ORGANIC FATS to keep your Veins SUPPLE and BUFFERED. (These all-VEGAN/RAW FOOD Diets, all the time can also make your cholesterol too low).

Too many people are taking STATIN Drugs LOWERING their CHOLESTEROL to DANGEROUS Levels! Yet, Doctors go on recommending this UNAWARE (or maybe they just do not care)? YOU need Cholesterol to make SEROTONIN (& many HORMONES). Good FOOD (fat) CURES for this? BUTTER, LECITHIN (both the Eggs and the Oil....*see Insite #54*), COCONUT CREAM/OIL. PHYSICAL CURE? UVB LITE. BLACK people have a higher requirement of Cholesterol (just like with most elements such as CALCIUM, SODIUM, MAGNESIUM and POTASSIUM). Meanwhile, high Cholesterol offers NEUROPROTECTION of the brain cells. In fact, CHOLESTEROL DEFICIENCY is one of the MAIN causes of ALZHEIMERS! This is why in many cases, the Cholesterol level goes up as we get OLDER! It is the BODYs way of Protecting us from the ravages of so-called FREE RADICALS/AGING. (see Insite# 0 & 54)

REVOLUTIONARY HEALTH INSITE #15: **INORGANIC SUGAR (from most BEVERAGES/SODAS/JUICES/LIQUORS)** is the number one cause of HEART ATTACKS. It produces a KHEMICAL/ALCOHOL that BURNS out those small, MICROSCOPIC muscles Deep in the Heart. This KHEMICAL destroys the protective SATURATED FAT of the Heart, getting into the MEAT/CORE of the HEART and then eroding it from the inside out. This form of HEART EROSION is hard to SEE or OBSERVE on an X-RAY/EKG—until its too late! (see Insite# 18 & 22)

REVOLUTIONARY HEALTH INSITE #16: **If a BABY is at least 6 POUNDS this is adequate for BIRTH during PREGNANCY even if they do not make it the full 10 months (or between 37-42 weeks).** A PREEMIE is just as NORMAL as a FULL TERM baby. Because being born at 34 weeks IS Full Term for some babies—while others can go as long as 44 weeks! Please be aware that the MOST important reason that babies are born small (outside of INHERITANCE)—is MAMA did not DRINK enough WATER and/or get enough FAT. Water and Fat are KRUCIAL to a developing child. Ample Water builds ample AMNIOTIC FLUID. Remember you are not only EATING for 2—you are DRINKING (and even THINKING for we caint discount the MIND-to-MIND connection) for 2 as well! Additionally, Water helps avoid the Dreaded PRE-ECLAMPSIA (HIGH BLOOD PRESSURE) so common in during PREGNANCY.
Meanwhile, FAT will help Grow the BRAIN/LUNGS of the baby. NEURONAL DEVELOPMENT will be affected which goes toward the SPINAL CORD and eliminating DISEASES like CYSTIC FIBROSIS, SPINAL BIFIDA and any other NERVE DEVELOPMENT MALFUNCTION. (see Insite# 158).

REVOLUTIONARY HEALTH INSITE #17: **PEACHES are NATURAL HORMONE REPLACEMENT THERAPY**. A whole SHIZZ load of PEACHES. In fact, you will be having a lot of SHIZZ for the TOILET so stay near it. However, the TOILET is what you likely need if you have ESTROGEN/HORMONAL issues. In other words, CONSTIPATION is a side-effect of ESTROGEN-related problems. Thus, rather than BIOIDENTICAL HORMONES feed your CELLS the FRUCTOSE SUGARS of SOUR/SWEET fruits like PEACHES, KIWI, POMEGRANATES, LEMONS, LIMES, ORANGES or VEGETABLES like SWEET POTATOES—all of which are good for MEN too (as they take on the MALE resonance when eaten by a MAN and the WOMAN resonance when eaten by her). All the key HORMONES are represented: ESTROGEN, TESTOSTERONE, ANDROGEN, DHEA, PROGESTERONE. (see Insite#9).

REVOLUTIONARY HEALTH INSITE #18: **The Recommended GLUCOSE LEVELS (of 80-120) is TOO DANGEROUSLY LOW for Black People**!! BLACK people (and People of Color) have a different STOMACH/PANCREAS FLORA/SYNTHESIS than WHITE PEOPLE *(some of which can be explained due to the amount of POST TRAUMATIC SLAVE DISORDER (Dr. Joy Leary) we live under ......also see Insite #0)!* Thus, we start CRAVING more SUGAR since at the 80-120 level we are NOT getting enough. Therefore, we start OVEREATING sugar and get DIABETES trying to CRUSH that CRAVING too quickly with SUCROSE: INORGANIC, SIMPLE REFINED TABLE SUGARS/CARBS (candies, cookies, juices, sodas, and so on). A range from 120-160 (even upwards of 200 with some individuals) would be more on point for the Black MAN/WOMAN. The MELANIN (ala CARBON) soaks up SUGAR more. Therefore, we need more GLUCOSE derived from FAT (via KETOSIS....which is when the body is operating off of its OWN fat stores) to begin with!! And not from Simple Sugars like TABLE SUGAR (SUCROSE) and REFINED SUGAR in CARBS like drinks, candies, and so on but more from FRUITS *(FRUCTOSE which have a lower GLYCEMIC level and do not JACK the BLOOD GLUCOSE up too fast).* The numbers that DOKTORS tell Black people they need to be is DESTROYING their VEINS as well as their PANCREASES. For those WHITE people with OBVIOUS mixed Blood, their GLUCOSE numbers are also skewed! (see Insite# 5, 6, 10 & 200).

REVOLUTIONARY HEALTH INSITE #19: **MEN SHOULD NOT EJACULATE (Nor should Women SQUIRT for the very same reasons)!** Unless its too help create a BABY. Otherwise, HOLD your SEED my bretheren of ALL Ethnicities! Because every time you BUST—is a LOSS of ZINC and BLOOD NUTRIENTS. This is one of the *main* reasons mean DIE earlier than WOMEN: they lose comparatively LARGE amounts of ZINC via EJACULATION over the years! As a result, their IMMUNITY suffers tremendously!! Low levels of ZINC affect HEART CONTRACTIONS resulting in INFARCTIONS/heart attack....for this reason men are at greater risk for HEART ATTACK than Women. Thus, it should be NO surprise that many men have Heart Attacks while EJACULATING during SEX! (they were already LOW on ZINC)! Likewise, ZINC is a very CRITICAL nutrient due to the fact that it is the MAN who PASSES on IMMUNITY (the MAMA passes on NERVE STRENGTH).

In fact, it is like giving Blood and OXYGEN (which is why we go to SLEEP). You have LOST Oxygen, Zinc and Blood—just to mention a few of the important NUTRIENTS (ZINC, SELENIUM, CHLOROPHYLL and IODINE being most important to keep stored in your TESTICLES......while the Mama needs to remain bonafide in IRON, OIL and B-VITAMINS). So STOP Busting so much! SEMEN is concentrated BLOOD, blood actually—which means it has more Nutrients in its SEED content than there is in, say, 6-12 pieces of FRUIT!! The reason for this is because whenever a MAN gets ready to EJACULATE, the body figures this is the time to MAKE BABY—and it PACKS the Best of what you got into that SEMEN—which would give the BABY the best start possible. Except, there is no Baby. You just BUSTING! This Literally KILLS You! Sets you up for PROSTATE and TESTICULAR issues. Only BUST when you intend to MAKE A BABY for the most part (there can be exceptions). Or BUST when you and the GODDESS are working on a HEALING WOMB Ritual for her (SPERM is good for the WOMB, especially, when it is produced by RITE Eating). Therefore, have an ORGASM, indeed (gotta CIR-CU-LATE) so that you RECYCLE your SEEDS like a TREE (which essentially Never DIES). You see, when you hold that SEMEN in--you actually REBUILD your SOIL (raw materials that make your Semen—you BOOST your RED BLOOD CELLS; help REPAIR your GENES and BONE MARROW because BLOOD CELLS are made in the REPRODUCTIVE SYSTEM<among other places>). RECYCLING is good for the COUNTRY—and its Good for YOU!

MALE EJACULATION or SQUIRTING (Female Ejaculation which seems to have become a RECREATIONAL SPORT these days) both are DANGEROOUS because they DRAIN the ENDOCRINE SYSTEMS of the MAN or WOMAN--and should be reserved for making BABIES (PROPAGATION rather than RECREATION). In fact, FEMALE EJACULATION while considered NORMAL by many SEXUAL ENTHUSIASTS (for its ORGASMIC POWER) is actually very Detrimental to the entire HORMONAL SYSTEM of the Woman-who LOSES a variety of her ESSENCES with this Practice (the same as a MAN who Ejaculates)....and is something that should be AVOIDED rather than ENCOURAGED. *(see Insite #85).*

REVOLUTIONARY HEALTH INSITE #20: **MEDITATION is MEDICATION so you do not need WEEDitation!** And has been for a time that may stretch back to 200,000 years ago including ancient NEW ZEALAND, AUSTRALIA, ASIA, INDIA, MIDDLE EAST, ATLANITS, LEMURIA, SHANGRILA and AFRIKA. The Great SAGES have been known to use MEDITATION for every known ILLNESS, SICKNESS and/or DISEASE. The SIDDIHIS of INDIA famously sit for HOURS to REGENERATE both MIND (SPIRIT....the CONSCIOUSNESS) and BODY (PHYSICAL....the ELECTRICITY in the body). MEDITATION is seriously underrated as a form of HEALING adjunct to ALL disease—even CANCER and AIDS!!

The Main reason that MEDITATION works is because it Stops GRAVITY (which exerts constant pressure) from PULLING on our BODIES—and thus our CELLS. Meanwhile, Meditation signals your BRAIN to SLOW down the CELLS—allowing them to work more efficiently—and CONSERVE ENERGY—which HEALS and EXTENDS LIFE (this is a built-in form of CELL REGENERATION, even STEM CELL REGENERATION—thereby building IMMUNITY)!! The MAHARISHI MAHESH YOGI was RITE to introduce the world to TRANSCENDENTAL MEDITATION (something everyone should learn/benefit from). When you allow your body to REST (via MEDITATION, SLEEP, as well as NAPPING, even)—you allow it to REGENERATE itself. And REGENERATION brings REPAIR(ATION) of a different kind. It's the kind of REPAIR that HEALS dis-ease, especially, ones that are STRESS-based such as HIGH BLOOD PRESSURE/HYPERTENSION, HEART-related, HEADACHES, EYEACHES, SINUS, BACK, FEET/ALIGNMENT issues, IRRITABLE BOWEL SYNDROME, STOMACH DISORDERS, CONSTIPTATION, SEXUAL DYSFUNCTION, ORGASMIC DIFFICULTIES (which has a lot to do with Breathing by the way), MENTAL DISTURBANCES, and so on. All you have to do is what my MAMA used to tell me: "GET SOMEWHERE AND BE QUIET" or more bluntly: "SIT YO ASS DOWN SOMEWHERE!" (see Insite #150).

REVOLUTIONARY HEALTH INSITE #21: **FAST YOUR LIFE AWAY!** And you will certainly LIVE LONGER. Fasting (along with UNDEREATING and general CALORIC RESTRICTION) removes TOXINS from the BLOODSTREAM allowing your CELLS to go back to their NORMAL size. Too much TOXEMIA swells up your BLOOD CELLS causing them to be SLUDGY and SLUGGISH. Normal size of a BLOOD CELL (said to be 7 MICRONS) means your BLOOD FLOW will be good. It means your HORMONAL FLOW will be good. Your LYMPH SYSTEM will be pristine (which is important because your LYMPHATIC SYSTEM is like the SEWER LINE in the body and needs to be CLEANED out, regularly). This translates to better IMMUNITY as well. And again, LONGER LIFE!

When you Decrease the need for your body to constantly Clean itself from EATING----you save VITAL fluids and tissues. And as well, INCREASE the ability of the body to REGENERATE its ORGANS, SKIN—even BONE.
Fasting will also REDUCE your WEIGHT. A very KEY point because most of us WEIGH too much for our BONE STRUCTURE—and that just means EXTRA Gravity and pressure on your Organs. The more pressure on your ORGANS the FASTER they WEAR out from STRESS. Fasting allows the BRAIN to REGENERATE its NEURONS much more quickly, too! This is crucial as you get OLDER—and tend to lose this ability without proper NUTRIENTS and REDUCTION of GRAVITY on the Brain. Well, Fasting encourages NEURONAL GROWTH/CONNECTIONS, MELANIN (CARBON) CREATION, MEMORY, SHARPNESS—leading to Bigger GLANDS, ie., HYPOTHALAMUS, PINEAL, PITUITARY and AMYGDALA—all which are ENDOCRINE affecting HORMONES, APPETITE, SEX DRIVE and AGING. These GLANDS can be knocked off line with a BAD Diet—yet, Fasting can bring

them back online and into ALIGNMENT. Remember: You can SLOW Life down if You FAST.

In study after study FASTING aka UNDEREATING aka CALORIC RESTRICTION extends and/or IMPROVES the HEALTH/LIFESPAN of Animals (from WORMS code named C. ELEGANS to MICE to ORANGUTANS). The key to all of this are the SIRTUIN GENES that are expressed when it picks up that the body is moving into a period of FAMINE. Thus, every time you FAST, you EXTEND the Life of your BLOOD CELLS due to the body releasing a hormone via the SIRTUIN GENETIC PATHWAY that SLOWS down their AGING. These CELLS are connected to the SIRTUIN GENES which CODE for LONGEVITY in the HUMAN PLANT.

Automatically, then, these so-called SIRT GENES (1-7) emit a KHEMICAL/HORMONE that slows down the CELLULAR CLOCK inside every cell that tells it when to DIE OFF. As a result your Cells last longer before DEATH (APOPTOSIS). They last longer and so do you.

This HORMONE is only emitted during times of FAMINE as a way to keep the SPECIES around. Often, the levels of REPRODUCTION are conserved as well—so that No FERTILITY is possible. However, NOT all the time does INFERTILITY happen. As well, Average BODY TEMPERATURE may drop, FAT STORES increase and so on with other BENEFICIAL physiologies happening.

REVOLUTIONARY HEALTH INSITE #22: **The PANCREAS is the most CRITICAL Organ if we want to Stop AGING (or at least SLOW IT DOWN)! For it controls how FAST we AGE—and has the most direct bearing on whether we obtain LONG LIFE!** The reason for this is that it controls the 2 KEY khemicals that affect ALL organs in the form of a SUGAR----GLUCOSE and GLUCAGON!

Glucose affects the SYMPATHETIC NERVOUS SYSTEM (or the STRESS System) and GLUCAGON affects the PARASMPATHETIC NERVOUS SYSTEM (or the REST System....and you want to REST as much as possible). PANCREATIC REST, for example, does NOT happen when you eat GRAINS (a CARBOHYDRATE) because they USE UP as much as 6 times the amount of PANCREATIC ENZYMES (fuel) than MEAT does to be DIGESTED!! Functioning like this produces Excessive GLUCOSE which acts like a POISON under these circumstances.

As a society we live off of GLUCOSE (carb) consumption! SUGAR this, Sugar that. Burning out our system with Glucose OVERLOAD! In fact, there was a recent study in which WORMS (called C. ELEGANS) were given extra GLUCOSE----and, as a result, their lives were SHORTENED by up to 20%! Thatz equal to about 20 years in human biology that they LOST! However, by the same token, when the INSULIN SIGNALING PATHWAY was SHUTDOWN—these WORMS lived LONGER than normal! The Insulin Signaling Pathway means ground zero for the functioning of the Pancreas. So its SUPER critical to EXTENDING your life past the 100 years of Age.

Many of us are losing MORE than 20 years off our lives when you add in all the other DETRIMENTAL things we are doing to our bodies......And it must be remembered that

CARBOHYDRATES, in general, are a HUGE part of our EATING—and thus continually EXHAUST the Pancreas which has to tirelessly supply DIGESTIVE juices to break down those CARBS! The Pancreas controls Carbohydrate METABOLISM with its PANCREATIC ENZYMES and INSULIN secretion. Here is the thing: a moderate amount of Pancreatic Enzymes and Insulin are okay inside the body. However, TOO MUCH and it drives up the level of GLUCOSE which in turn revs up the SYMPATHETIC NERVOUS SYSTEM and the HORMONES that supports it: CORTISOL & ADRENALINE----and this BURNS out not only your Pancreas--your other Organs inclusive of the LIVER and KIDNEYS suffer as well! This is what causes RAPID AGING, leading to so-called NATURAL DEATH!! Thus, KILL ya Pancreas—KILL YOURSELF!

So you can see that from the standpoint of DAILY living—your PANCREAS is the most IMPORTANT, CRITICAL Organ in the Body! NO ORGAN is more important than the PANCREAS for ensuring a LONG LIFESPAN. NOT ONE!!!! Every time you eat you affect your Pancreas which has to put in the most work. Thus, should make it clear to all of us then how important a strategy it is to FAST, periodically (1-2 days out of every 10-12 days is good). This way you give your PANCREAS a much needed REST. The less you have excessive GLUCOSE flowing in your BLOOD—the LONGER you will live! It can not get any simpler than that! *(see Insite 5, 6 & #18).*

REVOLUTIONARY HEALTH INSITE #23: **Black People are SALTY people! Yet, we do not eat enough SALT!** The RITE kind of SALT, that is. Like with SUGAR, most of our SALT /Sodium intake is INORGANIC, PROCESSED/REFINED (via CARBOHYDRATES) which INJURES our VEINS. However, a good, ORGANIC LIQUID Salt like FRUIT SALT (from LEMONS, LIMES, GRAPEFRUITS, ORANGES) contains all the ELEMENTAL salt, LITHIUM, IODINE and CALCIUM (aka known as VITAMIN C by me) one needs; or alternatively, HIMALYAN PINK SEA SALT which contains 72-something-odd VITAL MINERALS also including IODINE, MAGNESIUM and other TRACE MINERALS—is just what we need (make sure you find the SEA SALT that does indeed contain IODINE <or buy LUGOLS or IODORAL as supplement>....because some do not). Then there is the Supplemental SUGAR called SUCANAT which contains actual MINERALS whereas plain, white Sugar does not—thus, it is a better choice of the two (it is Less REFINED).

The FRANKENMEDS (doctors) have taken BLACK PEOPLE off salt—when we need it most in todays society, especially, with the STRESS levels we live under!! SALT alleviates STRESS and feeds the entire NERVOUS SYSTEMS and the BONES (preventing OSTEOPOROSIS)—and who is more stressed out in AMERIKA than Black People? Anyway, what they are calling HIGH BLOOD PRESSURE is not because SODIUM (salt) is bad; rather it is because most people are DEHYDRATED *(see Insite #26 and #32)* and the SODIUM in the Blood can not get into the CELLS without adequate WATER (hydration) and thus it BUILDS UP in the Bloodstream! Yet. It is NOT the SODIUM that is the Problem. It is the LACK of water! Meanwhile, Doktors go on prescribing YOU med-i-sins that your body can not use—and which also

DESTROY your VEINS! (then they say you DIED of High Blood Pressure because your Veins gave out)!

So we CRAVE salt but we do not GET ENOUGH salt!! NO SALT. NO SPARK. For Salt is the FIRE of the NERVOUS SYSTEM, indeed, of the ENTIRE body—thus, we need to act like PROMETHEUS and STEAL back the FIRE! Lack of Salt contributes greatly to CHRONIC FATIGUE (no fire), INSOMNIA (no spark to create SEROTONIN and LITHIUM both crucial HORMONES which help you SLEEP/RELAXES your NERVES), HEADACHES, OSTEOPOROSIS (SALT BUILDS BONES!----after all, CALCIUM <which is VITAMIN C> is----a SALT, one of the 4 major CELL SALTS). Lack of SALT is one reason why so many WOMEN have BAD ATTITUDES (not saying its you—but you know who you are or you know who im talking about). They are not getting enough SALT for proper HORMONE FORMATION (which affects MOODSWINGS). Drinking the Juice of LEMONS/LIMES is a great regular regimen. Additionally, your TEETH and GUMS will thank you (remember the case of SCURVY back in the day? It was LIMES that saved those sailors....why? VITAMIN C also known as CALCIUM because Vitamin C is simply CALCIUM! They are really one and the same)!!

Furthermore, SALT (like URIC ACID in Meat) is a Supreme ANTIOXIDANT and a chemical that PRESERVES and encourages the LONG LIFE of your BLOOD CELLS. It is a good reason BLACK PEOPLE have the capability to live so long, we have a Higher SODIUM content in our bodies (enhanced even more by MELANIN).

REVOLUTIONARY HEALTH INSITE #24: **INSOMNIA (and many other DIS-EASES) can be CURED by SLEEPING According to your BODY WEIGHT (and your CIRCADIAN RHYTHM).** In general, the SMALLER you are the LESS sleep you need; while the BIGGER you are the MORE sleep you need. Thus, a smaller person may need to stay awake 24-48 hours in a row before they can SLEEP comfortably and DEEPLY. While a Bigger person may only be able to stay up a maximum of 12-18 hours before requiring more sleep. Recall I mentioned how important MEDITATION/REST/NAPPING is for REGENERATION. Thus, how about this? You can SLEEP many DISEASES away!

That would make a great COMMERCIAL:
"I slept through TUBERCULOSIS and PSORIASIS. They were gone when I woke up!"

Diseases like CHRONIC FATIGUE can be remedied with 12-36 hours of proper DEEP sleep, depending on the severity. We SHALLOW BREATHE—and we SHALLOW SLEEP as well. We do not Breathe Deep enough nor do we Sleep deep enough, either. What the FRANKENMEDS (doctors) call DELTA SLEEP is STILL not deep enough. We are disturbed too much as we struggle to get to the sleep stage that would truly REGENERATE our CELLS!

Part of the Sleep problem is that EVERYBODY has a different sleep CYCLE. Often this difference is just by degrees—yet it makes a HELL of a difference! Millions of people can not get enough DEEP, SLEEPFUL rest in 8 hours. Some of you may need 10-12 or even 15 hours to feel REGENERATED! Some even a whole 24 hours of DEEP SLEEP may be required to COME BACK TO LIFE--or even YEARS as the case may be in instances of a COMA!! *(What I call the SLEEP of the DEAD which could require you remain in a COMA for as long as 10-20 years even in order for your body to HEAL properly)!!*

However, on the SHORTER side of things: this could simply require you stay up 24-48 hours straight—until you are DEAD TIRED! Then, CRASHING into bed! It is the only way you will be able to get the type of sleep you need! You do not want any DREAMS when you sleep (which is RESTFUL sleep—yet not deep REGENERATIVE sleep). You do not want to Remember ANYTHING about sleeping. You want to be COMPLETELY dead to the world when you are sleeping for REGENERATION. Every time you sleep! That is the type of sleep you NEED. That is when you gain NEW cells. That is when you HEAL for REAL! Because for you and many millions more LIKE you—8 hours is simply NOT enough sleep!!

Conversely, some of you may need only 1-4 hours sleep—and you are good. Because it was DEEP! And DEEP is the KEY in all of this. You have to find your CIRCADIAN RHYTHM so you can SLEEP DEEP. Sleep hard. You have to sleep with NO dreams. Dreams are a disturbance to DEEP SLEEP. In fact, anything that disturbs your DEEP SLEEP is a PROBLEM! Whether it be somebody BANGING on your DOOR, LOUD MUSIC----or DREAMS! Its all SLEEP DISTURBANCE and SLEEP DEPRIVATION. And it will/can make you SICK. CHRONICALLY FATIGUED. DEPRESSED. COMA and AUTO IMMUNE-prone. In short, all kinds of HEALTH issues from LACK of SLEEP. You are not SICK. You are SLEEPY!

Therefore, find out what your Sleep pattern is and you will HEAL a number of bodily issues that may be affecting you at this time. Being off of your CIRCADIAN RHYTHM is a form of SLEEPING SICKNESS or SLEEPING DISEASE brought on by this never sleep, 24—hour society.

Once you locate your CIRCADIAN RHYTHM and see that you are more of a DAY than a NITE person or vice-versa....then, your schedule has to be adjusted accordingly (even to taking a different job or work shift). Once you find your Rhythm, you will Sleep much better. Add LECITHIN to your eating (Eggs and/or the Liquid since this Nutrient helps the BRAIN form NEURONAL CONNECTIONS), and it will be even better. CIRCADIAN RHYTHMS determined by our BIOLOGICAL (INTERNAL) CLOCKS are CHANGING all over the world, affecting SLEEP PATTERNS. The HUMAN is starting to Sleep LESS and LESS with regular periods of staying AWAKE 24-48 hours.

Also adding NAPS is a very effective strategy (learning to sleep in SPURTS rather than long 8 hour blocks of time may be yet another method that works best for you) in completing your True RESTING/REGENERATIVE PHASE. Schedule naps regularly as part of your SLEEP CYCLE. Alternating the AMOUNT/LENGTH of time you SLEEP is also effective (4 hours one nite, 6 hours another nite. Its better to Sleep SHORT rather than LONG, thus averaging 4-6 hours is better than averaging 8 hours of sleep or more). We sleep TOO MUCH as a rule! The body needs to be ACTIVE. However, when you REST well, understanding that is also MEDITATION, NAPPING, WALKING, SITTING—simply getting somewhere and being MOTIONLESS is Rest too! Exceptions may be necessary such as SLEEPING extended periods (as mentioned above) on the order of 10-12 hours or more as a form of HEALING.

REVOLUTIONARY HEALTH INSITE #25: **GRAINS are DANGEROUS—and should be outlawed (and SUGAR too)!** They should be eaten in extreme moderation (if at all). The human digestive tract and its GUT BACTERIA still has not had time to get used to the KHEMICAL breakdown of GRAINS. Sure, grains have been around for about 10,000 years—but that is like 2 years in DIGESTIVE TRACT time! It is hard for the body to deal with breaking down grains in the GUT. Grains are an ultra processed food. Plus, they are THICK, STARCHY and full of indigestible FIBER and PHYTIC ACID that BINDS (clings to) VITAMINS/MINERALS in your Digestive Tract—and pulls them out during ELIMINATION (and pulls out the protective MUCUS in the Track). If you need FIBER, better to eat more natural grains: LEGUMES (certain beans like LENTILS—although, in moderation). Most of your HEALTH issues, especially, AUTOIMMUNE ones, such as CELIAC, FIBROMYALGIA, LUPUS, YEAST INFECTIONS are all Grain-related. Furthermore, the GLUTENS in grains generate a number of different ALLERGIC reactions from the body, causing enormous loads of HISTAMINE release. Histamines are what your body uses to cause you all of those ALLERGIES (ie., sniffles, even ANAPHALYTIC SHOCK)! The worst problem of grains is that they produce too much GLUCOSE in the BLOOD, causing the BLOOD SUGAR levels to remain ELEVATED for too long. It does not help that most of the Grains that we eat are from REFINED CARBOHYDRATES (WHITE BREAD, WHITE FLOUR, NOODLES, PASTA) which is metabolized into ALCOHOL (sugar and toxic ETHANOL)—that causes ORGAN, THERMAL FATIGUE, BURNING them out! And SUGAR *(see Insite #200)* is MURDER on the body! Just by eating GRAINS you can get (NON-ALCOHOL) CIRRHOSIS of the LIVER! (and you may have never even touched a drop of ALCOHOL/WHISKEY)!!

Civilizations that have tried to exist primarily on GRAINS have DIED OUT; or had STUNTED/DEFORMED Growth or SHORTENED lives: MAYANS, AZTECS, INCAS, OLMECS primarily, however, this can be seen around the world for any ETHNIC groups when you look at the ANTHROPOLOGICAL FOOD RECORDS. A wholly GRAIN-BASED Diet can not support a PEOPLE without terrible SICKNESSES and DEATH. Yes, Grains can be a PART of the FOOD SUPPLY (although in small amounts), yet must not be the MAIN food supply. Keep GRAINS to a MINIMUM!!

Indeed: The Moment our DIETS changed overwhelmingly--roughly 7,000-10,000 years ago during the NEOLITHIC PERIOD--in favor of More INSULIN-INDUCING CARBOHYDRATES (Grains) instead of more GLUCAGON-INDUCING PROTEINS & FAT (Meat and to a lesser degree: Vegetables and Fruits)--our LIFESPANS were CUT SHORT! (see Insite #22).

REVOLUTIONARY HEALTH INSITE #26: **The BODY needs HALF YOUR WEIGHT in OUNCES of WATER (however, sometimes this amount needs to be LESS....<see below>)!** As a people we do not drink enuff water: *We are DYING out because we are DRYING out!*

As a RULE, you use up about 64 ounces or half your weight in ounces of water everyday just thru daily living. The AMOUNT over and beyond half your weight in ounces depends on how much/often you EAT. And what you eat. EVERYTHING you do in your body is INFLUENCED by the Presence of WATER!! Therefore, even before FOOD you should be thinking about Water: 1-2 hours BEFORE you eat, drink water; WHILE you are eating, SIP water; and 30 mins-1 hour AFTER you are done eating, DRINK WATER!!

If you have eaten Lots of PROCESSED/REFINED Foods? Load up on the water! Have you eaten lots of FRUITS/VEGETABLES? Not as much water. Plenty of MEAT? Drink up plenty. Lots of GRAINS? Hopefully not, however, if so: Drink up again and again! Are you ACTIVE? More water? You OBESE? Hell of a lot of water! And so it goes.

Your Water amount depends on your LIFESTYLE. However, one point is CLEAR as Water! If you want your body CLEAN and FREE of TOXEMIA you need ample water. If you want help with your CELLS repairing themselves, you need ample water. The MEMBRANE around your cells need water—because that LIQUID is absorbed from the LYMPHATIC SYSTEM into the FAT CELLS where it is used for whatever needs to be done to that LINING/MEMBRANE. The membrane on the cell can wear away—thus, eroding your FILTER. Water along with FAT helps to MAINTAIN the MemBRANE!

What kind of water is best? DISTILLED. The argument some make that DISTILLED WATER takes the MINERALS shows IGNORANCE! *NOTE: they give BABIES Distilled Water to drink in the HOSPITALS. If it was so terrible to drink it, why then give it to babies whose Immune Systems are already at Risk? Furthermore, your CELL WATER is made via DISTILLATION! Thus DRINK the water that already has a natural, MOLECULAR and MAGNETIC AFFINITY for your BLOOD CELLS!*
Letz be clear: ANY water will take minerals out of your body! So its MISLEADING to say DISTILLED WATER will do so. What they DO NOT tell you, however, is that because of its Strong ELECTRICAL CHARGE----Distilled Water has the Highest MAGNETISM of any water—which means that AFTER your body is FLUSHED----and you then put, for instance, SEA SALT in your DISTILLED WATER—it has the best ability of any water for ATTRACTING minerals INTO your Cells (rather than OUT of them); and in the process—generating even MORE energy! (exactly what you need)!! This means Increased HYDROELECTRICITY (as the body heavily Hydroelectric) for you which translates into a sorta NUCLEAR POWER.

And for even BETTER results—you can BOOST the POWER of Distilled Water. Simply, BOIL it. Let it kool. Then Transfer it to GLASS BOTTLES. Add SEA SALT, BAKING SODA (non-aluminum like BOB RED MILLS brand) or ACV (apple cider vinegar). Another option: you can BOIL your TAP WATER which forces any TOXIC elements to the bottom (they use this technique in many indigenous/outback countries among the people to insure SAFE water. They simply BOIL it….works for them and it will work for you, too)!
NOTE: Very often the amount of water you drink needs to be LESS than HALF your WEIGHT in Ounces because it can be hard on your BLADDER. This is why this figure is just an AVERAGE. Somedays you should average LESS than HALF, drinking instead 25% of your weight. And eating more WATERY FRUIT in its

place! One can DRINK too much Water as well as TOO LITTLE as well. Vary your Water according to your ACTIVITIES that day. DO NOT just drink HALF your weight every, single day. On other days, drink more than HALF your weight (again based on your activities).

My other choices for WATER would be SPRING and/or WELL WATER. If you can ever find a highly, REPUTABLE source. Otherwise, stick with DISTILLED.

REVOLUTIONARY HEALTH INSITE #27: **The True Nature of ONIONS and GARLIC!** Onions are the most POTENT, natural ANTIBIOTIC you will find (really PROBIOTIC is the rite word because ANTIBIOTIC is like saying against life; while PROBIOTIC is like saying FOR LIFE). Onions mimic the WHITE BLOOD CELLs action. Thus, it helps FORTIFY the IMMUNE SYSTEM (the LYMPHATIC SYSTEM proper). Lay an ONION POULTICE on a SORE to HEAL it. Got a COLD/FLU? Drink a shot of Onion Juice (that is about 2 ounces). Got PNEUMONIA/RESPIRATORY issues? Drink Onion Juice and POMEGRANATE juice together. Got a STAPH INFECTION/MERSA? Pour Onion Juice over it. RABIES BITE? Onion juice.

No joke. ONIONS are truly Healing MEDICINE. In fact, it is probably the best NATURAL MEDICINE there is!! When it comes to KILLING off BACTERIA, GERMS or VIRUSES—in short, turning your Immune System around—you want the POWER of Onion!

GARLIC, while powerful as well, is best used as a SALVE on the SKIN to prevent INFECTION/RE-INFECTION/INFLAMMATION like with BABIES/OLD PEOPLE who Immunity has been affected. Maybe a person has BURNS. Then, make that GARLIC into a GARLIC POWDER and DUST the persons skin to give them IMMUNITY via the skin. Now, it can work in other ways, but it works best as a SALVE/POWDER.

In essence, you want to use the Onion INTERNALLY and the Garlic EXTERNALLY. Thatz how they work best together—and you get the MOST out of each.

CANCER RECIPE: *Mixing ONION JUICE with BAKING SODA is a great CANCER Healing recipe!! Make it into a PASTE. Swallow 2 tablespoons. 1-2 hours later drink 8 ounces of DISTILLED*

WATER. COLD. Of course, you must ADJUST the rest of your EATING too!

REVOLUTIONARY HEALTH INSITE #28: **At one time, we had No STOMACH or SMALL INTESTINE (going back past 2 million years ago before we started eating MEAT and PLANTS)!** This is due to us SURVIVING off of the ENERGIES of the SUN only (aka SOLARIANS)! And simply BREATHING in the RAYS of the GREAT LITE (BREATHARIANS). Thus, the SOLAR PLEXUS or said another way: SUN CENTER (plexus). Both of the STOMACH and the SMALL INTESTINE are only Recent ADAPTATIONS into the DIGESTIVE TRACT proper. Previously, there was ONLY the LARGE INTESTINE! It did the job of both the SMALL INTESTINE and STOMACH because it has way more SURFACE AREA than the SMALL INTESTINE, and thus about 6 times the ABSORPTION POWER! (after all, it is where WASTE is stored). However, as Wo/Man DE-EVOLVED s/he got a STOMACH and SMALL INTESTINE to DIGEST FOOD!

EVOLUTIONARILY speaking, it went like this: SUNLITE! (SOLARIAN) And then later, AIR (BREATHARIAN), then WATER (LIQUIDARIAN), then FRUITS (FRUITARIANS), VEGETABLES (VEGETARIAN), MEATS (MEATARIAN), GRAINS (GRAINARIANS) (and lastly the PROCESSED/REFINED FOODS we eat now!!—REFINARIANS...lol!).

Actually, eating SOLID FOOD is the LOWEST form for HUMANS to get FUEL. Furthermore, Solid Food mostly only gives us FIBER----NOT----ENERGY/FUEL as much. We get most of our Energy from the 2 NUTRIENTS that causes us to live the SHORTEST without them----OXYGEN aka PRANA aka LIVE PHOTONS and HYDROGEN aka HEAT aka SOLAR RAYS aka SUN RAYS. And not FOOD! Eating Solid Foods is a TRADE-OFF as it causes us such problems as SICKNESS, AGING/SHORT LIFE SPANS, and so on---due to taking a hell of amount of energy to process!! This promotes DISEASE. And THIS is the MAIN reason we have such a relatively long DIGESTIVE TRACK (compared to most CARNIVOROUS ANIMALS for example, however, not as long as most HERBIVOROUS ANIMALS). It is so that SOLIDS can have ENOUGH TIME to be DIGESTED properly—and so that proper ASSIMILATION can take place. Thus, being OMNIVOROUS, we have EVOLVED a Digestive Track between the length of CARNIVOROUS and HERBIVOROUS animals.

Conversely, 100% MEAT-EATING ANIMALS who Eat ALL raw meat ALL the time have short Digestive Tracks and do not live as long (in human years) or they AGE 2wice as fast! A short Digestive (mostly raw), Meat-eating Track (as opposed to LIQUID-EATING) equals a Short Life Span. This is because in order for the MEAT/FOOD to be really digested it takes about 10 times the amount of HCA (HYDROCHLORIC ACID aka HCL) than a HUMAN has. And it is all this ENERGY spent processing such an ELEMENT as RAW MEAT (and POISONS, TOXINS in the meat) that adds WEIGHT to the Digestive Track and Takes YEARS OFF the life of the Animal. It AGES them much Faster than HUMANS! *Altho, in the Transition to RAW EATING—a certain amount of MEAT-eating is necessary (however, no more than 1-4 ounces, perhaps, every 4-10 days, extending that time further apart as the body becomes more adept at going without Meat). Also this is what SHORTENS the lives of those who eat Meat: they eat TOO MUCH meat, upwards of 2.5 times their weight is eating meat. And thatz WAY too much URIC ACID that will be produced on such a DIET!!*

Your DIGESTION is a DELICATELY BALANCED operation that hinges on HOW LONG foods stay in your LARGE INTESTINE; or whether or not food gets processed quickly/properly enough in/thru the SMALL INTESTINE. If you are having problems with DIGESTION there is a good chance you are EATING foods that fall under one of these two categories. And is now causing

DISEASE. For example, DIVERTICULITIS or FECAL IMPACT (oil and hot water are the cure.

You must overstand that you live in a DIFFERENT time now. And to insist on eating as a HERBIVORE will cause the ATROPHY of your DIGESTIVE TRACK! It will PROLAPSE (fall, become longer as it stretches) to fit that of an ANIMAL who survives off PLANTS ONLY! Except for one thing: YOU are not such an ANIMAL!

REVOLUTIONARY HEALTH INSITE #29: **Drinking your URINE (even SEMEN or BLOOD may be necessary) to get well!** Drinking your own URINE or SEMEN is always in order (as a very LAST RESORT EFFORT)—if thatz what it takes to HEAL. Sometimes a situation could call for just that. Remember this: As the ANCIENTS showed us—EVERYTHING in your ENVIRONMENT represents a POTENTIAL, HEALING modality for the body proper. Including your OWN body fluids! Your URINE contains STEM CELLS.

The thing is knowing WHEN to drink your Urine. URINE DRINKING is best done when the Urine is CLEAR! Thus drink a lot of water prior to drinking urine wherever/whenever possible. So that the Urine is CLEAN and clear. Rather than Yellow or even light Yellow. Sometimes it may need to be YELLOW—or KLEAR. They both have different functions depending on ILLNESS. In general, you drink it as more YELLOW urine when your SICKNESS is more about your BLOOD, ie., LOW WHITE BLOOD CELL COUNT, LUPUS, SJROGENS, ANEMIA. Catch the FIRST urine in the morning after counting about 6 seconds. Drink this with a few ounces of LEMON JUICE/ACV. In connection with appropriate DIETARY changes—drinking your own URINE boosts your COMPLETE BLOOD COUNT!

On the other hand, CLEAR urine is the ELIXIR of choice as a SALINE SOULUTION when you are trying to replace ELECTROLYTES or you are DEFICIENT in MICRONUTRIENTS like SODIUM, POTASSIUM, SELENIUM, ZINC—all of which can be implicated in diseases like KIDNEY DISEASE, EDEMA and so on. Clear Urine also helps clean your LYMPH which is just as important as your BLOOD. The LYMPH carries nutrients and bathes the blood, in effect, providing STERILIZATION to a degree. DETOXING affects your LYMPHATIC CIRCULATION. And URINE is part of that DETOXIFICATION process—made in the LABORATORY—inside YOU! Inside your KIDNEYS (which are a PETRI DISH<also the BLADDER>) of the body.

REVOLUTIONARY HEALTH INSITE #30: **ACTIVATED CHARCOAL, LECITHIN and CLAY are Superior ways to DETOX from DRUG ADDICTION!** Why? Because ACTIVATED CHARCOAL contains CARBON/ MELANIN *(see LECITHIN below).* This makes it attractive to the MELANIN SITES which influence ADDICTION. Carbon is a conductor and an ABSORBER. When it comes into contact with a drug, say, NICOTINE in CIGARETTES or THC in WEED—it CLINGS to it chemically. Your BRAIN reads this as a GOOD FEELING, and thus, wants to REPEAT the process. Therefore, when the NICOTINE/THC is not around you have a CRAVING. This is ADDICTION. This is the release of too much DOPAMINE which deals with PLEASURE and REWARD as well as AGGRESSION. At any rate, you need to replace the ADDICTIVE KHEMICAL with something else just as attractive (magnetic) to the MELANIN for CLINGING. This in turn will help you pull away from the CRAVING of the DRUG. Thus, your BEST BET is ACTIVATED CHARCOAL. In fact, ACTIVATED CHARCOAL is a standard treatment for people who have been POISONED. And basically, you have been: Only via NICOTINE, THC or even ALCOHOL!!

The ACTIVATED CHARCOAL and/or CLAY is used to DRAW OUT the Poison from your BLOODSTREAM, NERVOUS SYSTEM/CEREBROSPINAL FLUID via the STOMACH, SWEAT, SALIVA, BOWEL MOVEMENTS, TEARS and so on. All pertinent FLUID EXTRACTIONS come into play. This is MAGNETISM at work. The Activated Charcoal or Clay is a stronger force than the KHEMICAL of the DRUGS you were taking. You TREAT/HEAL yourself by taking SMALL amounts over time. And start REDUCING the amount of the DRUG (Cigs/Weed).

Also take organic SUGAR/SWEETS (SUCANAT, MOLASSES, for example) because you will CRAVE the taste of SUGAR. Also FRUITS like PEACH, APRICOT, MANGO, PLUM, NECTARINE (Note: if necessary, you can also eat CHOCOLATE ICE CREAM/SHAKE or drink CHOCOLATE MILK or HOT CHOCOLATE). Standby for MASSIVE BOWEL MOVMENTS as you begin to CLEANSE/DETOX/FLUSH your SYSTEM. You may also VOMIT! But this is all in the service of ELIMINATING that POISON/DRUG. The SUGAR Binds/Clings to the AC and helps for a faster elimination, also acting as a BUFFER. *(see DICK GREGORYs book COOKING WITH MAMA NATURE).* You can make your own ACTIVATED CHARCOAL by burning TOAST, PEANUTS and so on. You can buy the CLAY online.

The other Key NUTRIENT for Detoxing off of DRUGS (COCAINE, CRACK, WEED, METH) is LECITHIN. Much needed for REPLACING the Brain Khemicals such as SEROTONIN, MELATONIN and DOPAMINE which are all instrumental in you being able to maintain WELL-BEING. This THICK oil is a precursor to these nutrients and helps the brain produce them in abundance. This in turn helps with your MENTAL in terms of DEPRESSION or BI-POLARISM. And it will allow your Brain to catch up the IMBALANCE that has been created by Doing the Drugs. In fact, LECITHIN may be the MOST effective Nutrient for DEPRESSION and SCHIZOPHRENIA *(see Insite #54).*

REVOLUTIONARY HEALTH INSITE #31: **FRUITS are simply edible HERBS!** From the field of BOTANY described as the RIPENED OVARY of a PLANT from Latin PLANTA meaning HERB. Thus, FRUITS are HERBS you can EAT. And they are the HERBS that can truly be used for the HEALING of the NATION *(with all Respects to DR. SEBI).* Furthermore, FRUITS are just simpler to deal with. We know them from eating and being around them all our lives. Plus, it is a lot easier to go to the store and buy an APPLE or LEMONS than say CASCARA SAGRADA for CONSTIPATION, for example. Less chance for CONFUSION.

In other words, whatever AILS you can be HEALED just as well with FRUITS as TRADITIONAL herbs. And they TASTE good! That never hurts. Additionally, they are not as DANGEROUS (allergies not withstanding). It is hard to OVERDOSE on ORANGES or POMEGRANATES. Yet, POMEGRANATES are the PERFECT food for EMPHYSEMA. Pomegranates can HEAL you of this LUNG DISEASE. GROUND UP a couple of APRICOT seeds and you got a great HERB for boosting your WHITE BLOOD CELL count. CUCUMBERS and/or BLUE BERRIES are good for your BLOOD and OXYGEN. The INSIDE of ORANGE PEELS are good for the CAPILLARIES (smallest veins in the body).

HERBS have a place, yes. But more as a last resort. Otherwise, as long as you have FRUITS, you have a ready made HERB available to you. This is not an attempt to DISCREDIT herbs. Only to BROADEN the definition so that we know better our healing options—and avoid confining ourselves to only thinking of TRADITIONAL HERBS for healing—and FRUITS only for EATING (or the occasional sweet snack).

Fruits are the HIGHEST foods possessing FOTON/LITE ENERGY (PHOTONS are one of the smallest, yet most powerful particles of an ATOM. It packs nuclear energy into the smallest amount of space!). It is the Ultimate PHOTON/FOTON FOOD. With the Highest VIBRATION. True MEDICINE.

REVOLUTIONARY HEALTH INSITE #32: **DEHYDRATION is one of those HIDDEN Diseases!** Constant THIRST is not just a sign of DIABETES *(see Insite #23 and #26).* It can also be a reflection of INTERNAL issues dealing with the PANCREAS, LIVER and SPLEEN, indeed, the STOMACH itself! In MOST cases of SICKNESS the MAIN, UNDERLYING Cause is LACK OF WATER!! Simple DEHYDRATION *(Dr. BATMANGHELIDJ was right)!* You may not be properly absorbing the 4 major CELL SALTS including CALCIUM, MAGNESIUM, POTASSIUM or SODIUM. These are the ELECTROLYTES. Thirst may simply be signaling a slite (not necessarily SERIOUS) malfunction. Constant Thirst is part of that FIRST LINE of DEFENSE that our bodies use to let us know that something is RONG with our HEALTH. It is like a lite on our car dashboard telling us to CHECK ENGINE; or signaling the RADIATOR is overheating or the OIL is low. SOULUTION? Drink HALF your WEIGHT in OUNCES of WATER as a start. And at least TWICE a week, make sure to drink 2 ounces of FRUIT SALT (in the form of LEMON juice); or take one-quarter teaspoon of SALT in 8-12 ounces of WATER.

The best WATER to drink is DISTILLED. HOT, distilled water at that. Like a TEA. Then, ROOM TEMPERATURE and COLD. In that order. The rule can be broken wherever you feel necessary which is always the overriding key to HEALTH. It may, in fact, be MEDICINAL for you to drink COLD WATER *(headache, for example, which cold water drank real fast can help with).*

REVOLUTIONARY HEALTH INSITE #33: **You have had the same BLOOD since you were Born! It simply has been RECYCLED (every 8.25 years=33.0 years, and thus CRUCIFIXION!! Or said another way: LIFE AT THE CROSSROADS preparatory to CHANGE!!) and CLEANSED by the LIVER, KIDNEYS, SPLEEN, HEART, LUNGS, STOMACH and LYMPH NODES.** All of which are FILTERING and PRODUCTION STATIONS (not just the LIVER). The HEELS and BONE MARROW as well get into the act of RECYCLING the Blood Supply. You may recall the HEEL PRICK done to detect BRAIN DEFECTS. Your BLOOD is a CONCENTRATED ACID and on the OILY side (its WATER content notwithstanding). The BLOOD inside your BONES—the BONE MARROW or BONE FAT, is indeed a FATTY, OILY tissue that is for EMERGENCY BLOOD, ie., TRANSFUSIONS or whenever RED BLOOD CELLS die off----more new ones are made inside the BONES as well as the previously mentioned bodily locations.

When doing a BONE MARROW TRANSPLANT, the MARROW should be taken from the HEEL (for an ADULT). The YOUNGER the RECEIVER of the Transplant is—the HIGHER UP the body you take the Marrow, indeed, going all the way up to the SKULL if the RECEIVER is a CHILD, especially, of 5-6 years of age. And only take the MARROW from the RECEIVER. If this is ABSOLUTELY not possible, use their BROTHER or SISTER closest in AGE and of the SAME SEX (preferably).

REVOLUTIONARY HEALTH INSITE #34: **BREATHHOLDING for 60-seconds can add 10 minutes to your life EVERY TIME you do it!** Every time you HOLD your BREATH you increase the ability of your BODY to change CARBON DIOXIDE into OXYGEN. Increasing your RED BLOOD CELLS (and the HEMOGLOBIN which is the OXYGEN carrying MELLAPROTEIN in the BLOOD CELL).

REVOLUTIONARY HEALTH INSITE #35: **FEED Your BRAIN These FOODS!** The BRAIN is known for its 3 major HOUSES: The REPTILIAN BRAIN, the LIMBIC BRAIN and the NEO CORTEX. And within these 3 HOUSES are 4 Major Sections: The FRONTAL LOBE, PARIETAL LOBE, OCCIPITAL LOBE and TEMPORAL LOBE. And ALL of these areas MUST receive the RITE amount of NUTRIENTS to be WHOLE. And more importantly, to FUNCTION at PRIME rate!

We know that the BRAIN is mostly WATER, FAT, SUGAR and SALT. It is said that at least 1/3rd is LECITHIN (OIL) by dry weight. With SUGAR and SALT comprising the remainder. Of course, other MICRONUTRIENTS figure into the mix as well, ie., COPPER and MERCURY (too much--and you get AUTISM).

At any rate:
The FRONTAL LOBE deals with LOGIC/REASONING. Thus, its PRIMARY FOOD (nutrient) is organic OIL (for DEVELOPMENT). Symptoms: if you cant think CLEARLY or make sense of things.

The PARIETAL LOBE deals with SPACE/PERCEPTION. Thus, its PRIMARY FOOD (nutrient) is organic SALT (i.e., SEA SALT). Symptoms: VERTIGO/DIZZINESS.

The OCCIPTAL LOBE deals with VISION/DEPTH PERCEPTION. Thus, its PRIMARY FOOD (nutrient) is organic MICRONUTRIENTS ala RETINOIC ACID/VITAMIN A (CODLIVER OIL/EFAs). Symptoms: EYESITE.

The TEMPORAL LOBE deals with TIME/EMOTIONS. Thus, its PRIMARY FOOD (nutrient) is TRYPTOPHAN, GLUTAMIC ACID (ie., contained in foods such as CHEESE, GRAPES, organic

SUGAR such as SUCANAT, certain DARK MEATS, FISH) all of which help to produce SEROTONIN, a Natural NEUROTRANSMITTER in the Brain which brings PEACE of MIND, QUIETUDE. Is known to INCREASE during MEDITATION, for example.
SYMPTOMS: DEPRESSION and so on. Hard DRUGS such as CRACK, COCAINE (even WEED to a degree) can UPSET your SEROTONIN Balance. And definitely REFINED FOODS can knock this BIOCHEMICAL out of BALANCE!

So in a constant Evolving CYCLE we have to make sure our BRAINS get the CORRECT (righteous) Nutrients to perform at OPTIMUM levels. Mix your MEALS up. And Eat ORGANIC, FRESH (and even RAW) foods. Eat for your GENDER TYPE. Eat for your BODY TYPE. Eat for your BLOOD TYPE. And certainly Eat for your ETHNIC TYPE. It all helps as your body turns FOOD MATTER into ENERGY that MATTERS. *(see Insite #30 and #54).*

REVOLUTIONARY HEALTH INSITE #36: **The Greatest ADVANCE in HEALING and CURING DISEASE was NOT Medicine—rather it was simply CLEANLINESS (HYGIENE)!** Simply, addressing UNSANITYARY conditions in and around the cities in which people lived was the MAIN strategy that STOPPED/PREVENTED so many diseases of the MODERN AGE! (recall the BUBONIC PLAGUE)—Thus, it was not WESTERNIZED MEDICAL TREATMENTS, VACCINES, POTIONS, PILLS and SURGERIES! It was basically just more people WIPING their ASSES and WASHING their HANDS!! And CLEANING UP their ENVIRONMENT is what Truly SAVED HUMANITY from becoming ZOOMANITY. *(see The RACIST WHITE BLOOD CELL DIAGNOSIS in my other book to follow).*

REVOLUTIONARY HEALTH INSITE #37: **The Body is Meant to AGE (slowly) and Not DIE for HUNDREDS if not THOUSANDS of Years! Perhaps, NOT AT ALL!** You are comparatively IMMORTAL. It is only society that convinces you of the DEATH URGE which shortens your life! If a TREE can live for 4,000 years—what of the UNIVERSEs supreme human tree? (The HUMAN PLANT)? At a minimum, you should live as long as your local backyard TREE (some of which have been around for 10 generations). The so-called SIRTUIN CELLS in your body are SELF-REGENERATING (provided they have the Rite NUTRIENTS/LIFESTYLE, ie., CARBON, FAT, WATER and FASTING*...<per the work of Dr. ALEX CARREL and LEONARD HAYFLICK—they Both were RITE>)!!* Just like STEM CELLS, BONE MARROW CELLS and of course, your LIVER CELLS (which completely Regenerate the Liver overnite aligning it with the Mythical life of PROMETHEUS whose liver was eaten daily by a VULTURE but regenerated itself nightly).

So Yes, we are meant to AGE. SLOWLY tho. Very SLOW. However, Not to DIE as we know it! The DEATH as we know it amounts to SUICIDE!!!! Thatz why we keep REINCARNATING—we do not get it. AGING is our DEATH. Therefore, we are to RECYCLE (our cells like a TREE recycles its LEAVES) – and become YOUNG again. However we do not because we do not put the RITE Foods into our body that ENABLES our CELLS to REGENERATE IMMORTALY!!
Learn to give up your DEATHYSTYLE for a righteous LIFESTYLE that will have you living an ETERNAL HEALTHY LONG LIFE!

REVOLUTIONARY HEALTH INSITE #38: **ORGASMS for WO(MEN) are Overrated!** You do not need one to enjoy LOVEMAKING. In fact, it is better NOT to orgasm. At all. Period. Just keep recycling that energy you build up during sex. And save it for the next or (much) later session. You want to BUILD UP to ALMOST orgasming. But do not. Keep that FIRE going the entire Lovemaking. But never ORGASM. This is one of the most HEALING techniques that can be used to HEAL a WOMANs WOMB!! And to bring Inner Equilibrium to her ORGANS because this sort of INJACULATION literally BATHES the ORGANS in PRANIC ENERGY (which is what keeps the CELLS alive). NON-ORGASMIC SEX also builds Discipline that affects other parts of your LIFE. This will HELP your WILL in every other part of your life. The FLESH will no longer be WEAK while the SPIRIT is strong. Both will BENEFIT. You STACK the Orgasms from SMALLER ones to LARGER ones like a REVERSE Pyramid. Then, at some point later in one of your LOVEMAKING sessions----RELEASE the ORGASM—with a PRAYER, COMMANDMENT or whatever else you decide to utter at that moment. Combine this with your EATING MAKEOVER for a more HOLISTIC approach and it will CHANGE your life. ORGASMS should be had in MODERATION!

REVOLUTIONARY HEALTH INSITE #39: **BABY DELIVERY METHODS are BARBARIC!** And Backwards. The normal range of 10 CENTIMETERS is NOT the end of the road for the child to come out. S/He may be taking the long road to come here and thus may not arrive here until 12 CENTIMETERS or 15, even 20 CENTIMETERS. You can not time MAMA NATURE! Every WOMANs body is DIFFERENT! (Fellas please remember this)! To Induce LABOR is to ROB a CHILD of their DEVELOPMENT time in the WOMB! At that point every last second counts! If the MAMA is in DANGER, thatz one thing. However, as long as the MAMA is having the usual CONTRACTION pains—she MUST be allowed to DILATE as wide as she NEEDS to for the Delivery of the child. As it stands now, current methods of Delivery are forcing our children out with their BARBARIC methods! A small woman, for example, may have to Dilate to damn near 20 centimeters to get that BABY out! But thatz her. Another woman may only need 8 centimeters. These FRANKENMEDS are messing up the BOND between MAMA and BABY even before the Baby gets here—altho the Mama and Child had an agreement prior on a spiritual level.

The FRANKENMEDS worry (needlessly) that Dilating too long, keeping the MAMA open like that can/will cause INFECTIONS. Not if they INCUBATE her!! However, in this RUSH-RUSH world of ours, they do not have time for that! The HORSEpital CREDO: Another woman needs to have her baby in 2 hours in the same delivery room—so do whatever to get that Mama out of here! Women are under TREMENDOUS STRESS to have their BABIES under Todays ABNORMAL delivery room setup. What we call a PREEMIE is not a Preemie. If the child is ready to be born at 8 months---then, its just READY to be born, dammit! All you have to do is keep the child INCUBATED for about another 4-6 weeks

S/HE continues to develop. Feed the NEWBORN the Mamas BREASTMILK. No PROBLEM.

In a HUMANE world, BABIES WOULD BE BORN IN WATER—and women would NOT have to get C-SECTIONS. All BABIES. I repeat, ALL BABIES must come thru the VAGINAL CANAL (if at all possible). The VAGINA can open as WIDE as it needs to for delivery. Even hips come out of SOCKETS; and the SPINE can STRETCH if necessary to have the child. The child LOSES vital IMMUNITY FACTORS (a la Bifido bacterium infantis and Bifido bacterium longum) when it is cheated out of VAGINAL BIRTH. C-Sections are FORCING them out TOO SOON!

The Main STRATEGY for a PREGNANT woman is to KEEP the SPINE LIMBER with BELLY DANCING, STRETCHING, WALKING (not running, please). This way, LABOR is LESS of a TRAUMATIC experience—and more of an ENJOYABLE one. The other Strategy to PREVENT BIRTH DEFECTS is to take PLENTY of OIL and WATER. You are not only Eating for 2, you are DRINKING (water) for 2 as well. The baby NEEDS that water to help build up its AMNIOTIC FLUID (affecting LUNGS), and Avoiding Pregnancy-related issues such as PRE-ECLAMPSIA (high blood pressure) and GESTATIONAL DIABETES. And the OIL helps the development of the BABYs brain while in the womb.

REVOLUTIONARY HEALTH INSITE #40: The **VEGAN/RAW FOODS/VEGETARIAN Diet is mostly a WHITE PERSONS Diet and is therefore UNSAFE for most BLACK PEOPLE due to BLOODTYPE (as well as ANCESTRY, ETHNICITY, LOCATION and METABOLIM....*see Insite #0)!*** Thus, under the current PLANETARY and ENVIRONMENTAL paradigm (stresses, pollutions, toxins, lead in the water, mental programming, food chemicals, alternating spins/vibrations of the planet, soil depletion and so on)—VEGETABLES can not Deliver enough BIO-AVAILABLE nutrients or minerals to the BLACK BODY! At least, NOT by themselves. They need to be combined with FRUITS, NUTS, SEEDS, DAIRY and MEAT. A LACTO-OVO VEGETARIAN diet which includes CHEESE, EGGS and BEEF (Grass-Fed Beef, for example) would be the better of the two.

The WHITE BLOODSTREAM has a more of a resonance for such a MONO DIET as RAW PLANT FOODS only. (Although this does not mean that even all of my WHITE BRETHEREN/SISTREN will be successful on it). As well WHITE People have a STOMACH ACID more suited to Eating RAW FOODS in general. Why? Again, GEOGRAPHICAL ANCESTRY and LOCATION codes their DNA more for this. With some PEOPLE OF COLOR, Of course, it can be done—but as a whole most People of Color NEED MEAT in varying amounts. The WHITE BLOODSTREAM has also evolved for these same reasons so that it contains more WHITE BLOOD CELLS on average as well.

Granted, to any of my WHITE BRETHEREN/SISTREN reading this—even many of you can not and SHOULD NOT be VEGANS either! For the exact same reasons. Mainly, because some of yawl are not as WHITE as you think you are – and likewise, your

STOMACH FLORA and Bloodstreams can not handle the DIGESTIVE efforts of RAW FOODS! (see Insite# 0).

REVOLUTIONARY HEALTH INSITE #41: **CELIBACY is just as necessary as SEX!** As a form of SELECTIVE SEX----CELIBACY is an ENLIGHTENING concept. Not done as the FUGGED UP, FASHIONISTA method of today which ISOLATES your SPIRIT from yourself. Yet, it is supposed to bring you closer to yourself (however, thatz the TRICKERY of MIND CONTROL....DOWN is UP and UP is DOWN)! Thatz backwards and our ancestors saw this with FIRST EYE AWARENESS.

Here is how CELIBACY can help you when you are on Rite FREQUENCY:
#1—when it is done as a result of TRAUMA (rape, molestation or other forms of sexual/physical abuse; real bad relationship breakups).
#2—For SHORT to LONG TERM purposes of RITUALISTIC HEALING to AFFIRM SELF.
#3—For Removing SICKNESS
#4—For EMOTIONAL recovery

In other words, CELIBACY is ANALAGOUS to and a FUNCTION of SEXUAL FASTING. And it should ONLY be Broken with SEX for the same reasons of SACREDNESS (ie., bringing a child into this DIMENSION that has indicated its readiness to come here; or maybe you need to accomplish something <this gets more into SEXUAL MAJICK>). Having SEX like this is as effective as any SACRIFICE (that the DIABOLICAL ONES perform). Indeed, it is a SACRIFICE. Anytime FLUID (SALVE for the woman; SEMEN for the man)—is used it is a POWERFUL act (even SPITTING).

Most of us, instead, are SLAVES to SEXUAL FASHION. Becoming a CELIBATE because it sounds good to say it—rather than for its TRUE healing purpose. Then, its certainly not good for the spirit under those circumstances. (Being CELIBATE when one should not be is just as DETRIMENTAL as being OVERLY ACTIVE in SEXUAL LIFESTYLE, ie., the same VENOMOUS CHEMICALS/HORMONES are RELEASED and therefore INJURIOUS to your ORGANS)!! As a True SEX FAST, however, CELIBACY is a BEAUTIFUL modality, one that starts at the ROOT CHAKRA and works upwards before re-entering into the arena of SACRED SEX. Rather than enter into CELIBACY for MISINFORMED reasons which can SPLIT you (when it should REJUVENATE you) we must honor the CYCLE of Celibacy only when its due. Strive for Balance in all with our LOVEMAKING or NON-LOVEMAKING.

Then too, it must not be forgotten that when you have NO SEX those Glands that are essential to HEALING your BRAIN can Self-Regenerate: PITUITARY, PINEAL and HYPOTHALAMUS are especially important to Emotional WELL-BEING. The HORMONES contained within your PITUITARY, for example, are RE-SUPPLIED and Built up to their prior levels. This helps bring you back to BALANCE and EQUILIBRIUM.

REVOLUTIONARY HEALTH INSITE #42: **The LAW of ATTRACTION has become a BOGUS MARKETING SCHEME** that TRAPS you in a CONSTANT cycle of DESIRE and DEGENERATION! And its PROPONENTS or AGENTS are more of these FALSE PROPHETS (PROFITS?) promising that you can GAIN the WORLD (as you LOSE your SOUL)! Do Not STRIVE for anything; rather KNOW that everything you NEED (not Desire) will find its way to YOU because that is the True LAW of MAGNETIZATION (rather than ATTRACTION).

There is nothing that you MUST do EXCEPT
live your LIFE as RIGHTEOUSLY as you can.
As OPENLY as you can.
As MODESTLY as you can
As UNAMBITIOUS as you can.
As SPIRITUALLY as you can.
With NO EXPECTATION of REWARD! Anything you STRIVE for you will NOT be able to KEEP. Anything that you WAIT for will be Yours for as LONG as you NEED it. The REWARD takes care of itself (just as PUNISHMENT does—this is KARMA—it is All PROGRAMMED into our DNA). These are the TRUE LAWS of this EXISTENCE that those who SEEK to CONTROL us with their PROVACTEUR PROFITEERS will not tell you about.

REVOLUTIONARY HEALTH INSITE #43: **By 2012 and BEYOND--the Amount of LITE your BLOOD CELLS can Absorb will determine your LONGEVITY!** We must overstand that our BLOOD CELLS (specialized ones call CRYPTOCHROMES) are essentially SOLAR PANELS that ABSORB the RAYS of the SUN (this is why our SKIN absorbs rays rather than DEFLECT it—it is a holdover from an EVOLUTIONARY period when we EXISTED solely thru TAKING LITE IN FROM THE SUN=PHOTOSYNTHESIS). However, after we DEGENERATED, we lost this ability to SURVIVE solely off SUN RAYS—yet, our CELLS retained this to the extent that we can still GAIN much energy from the SUN. And when used correctly, we can REGENERATE the BODY and thus our HEALTH. The more one increases this ability to ABSORB and TRANSMUTE Sun Rays—the LONGER life will be. Thus, it is CRITICAL to drink WATER that has been CHARGED by the Sun (as well as drink HOT WATER w/LEMON JUICE), SUNBATHE (during SUNRISE and SUNDOWN; and occasionally at HIGHNOON). This will put your CELLS in a Higher SPIN CYCLE which enables them to ABSORB the SUNRAYS more efficiently.

Likewise, with the MOON. Drinking MOONwater, BREATHING deep at FULL MOONS. Exercising, Walking during the FULL MOON are all important. LOVEMAKING at FULL MOON is crucial too. Eating VEGETABLES (some technically are FRUITS) that MATURE at NITE are likewise an important EATING strategy (ie., ONIONS, TOMATOES, POTATOES, GREEN PEPPERS, and so on).

REVOLUTIONARY HEALTH INSITE #44: **The FRANKENMEDS long ago figured out that the BRAIN could be Completely RE-WIRED aka NEUROGENESIS (or more ominous: BRAINWASHING) simply by MANIPULATING the FOOD SUPPLY!** So here we stand on the brink of EXTINCTION because our MOUTHS have gotten us into trouble again! 12 NERVES coming straight out of the CRANIUM, all leading to the TONGUE should be a sober REMINDER how easy it is to STEAL the MINDS of a PEOPLE through TASTE alone! (see Insite# 52).

REVOLUTIONARY HEALTH INSITE #45: **A DIET that is just RIGHT for SOMEBODY ELSE may be totally RONG and even dangerous for YOU!** Rather than EATING by the BOOK or whatz being HYPED (such as a VEGAN/VEGETARIAN/RAW FOODIST/FRUITARIAN Diet)--continue to eat food that RESONATES with YOU (be it PLANT-based or more MEAT-based)—as long as its BALANCED, LIVE, WHOLE, CLEAN, ORGANIC and in general of HIGH QUALITY! This way, you can PLAN your EATING around a variety of FOODS that include MEAT (that the majority of us need....again, despite the hype & the books that are AGAINST eating Meat)!

REVOLUTIONARY HEALTH INSITE #46: **In STUDIES with both ANIMALS (and PRISONERS), those kept under constant LIGHTS developed a wide range of ILLNESSES** including CHRONIC FATIGUE, DIARRHEA, ULCERS, HEADACHES, AUTOIMMUNE DISEASES & MENTAL PSYCHOSES. This Mimics the current Industrialized, constantly lit, 24-hour Society we live in today and how it affects our HORMONES. WE ARE TIRED and EXHAUSTED and dont even realize how much. We have run our SYMPATHETIC NERVOUS SYSTEM into the ground at the expense of activating our PARASYMPATHETIC NERVOUS SYSTEM which can SAVE our Health. (see Insite #24)

REVOLUTIONARYHEALTH INSITE #47: **The Moment our EATING HABITS changed overwhelmingly in favor of More INSULIN-SIGNALING CARBOHYDRATES (Grains) instead of more GLUCAGON-INDUCING PROTEINS & FAT (from MEAT)--our LIFESPANS were CUT SHORT**, as we became DISEASE-ridden with all manner of life-taking illnesses including INFERTILITY, RETARDATION, DEFORMITIES and AUTO-IMMUNITY. This contributed heavily to the EXTINCTION of whole cultures! This came about with FARMING/AGRICULTURE (the NEOLITHIC PERIOD, approx. 7,000-10,000 years ago). (see Insite #22 and 25).

REVOLUTIONARY HEALTH INSITE #48: **As a RULE look for PROBIOTICS that contain B. LONGUM and B. INFANTIS CULTURES. These are EMBYONIC CULTURES meaning they were present at your BIRTH to give you IMMUNITY and are the strongest Natural BACTERIAL CULTURES (also obtained in MAMAs BREASTMILK).** We LOSE them from our GUT FLORA due to EATING HABITS (Sugar and Refined Carbs mostly...however, Drugs, Alcohol, Prescription Meds will deplete them too). Yet, they can be REPLACED with a PROBIOTIC FOOD (ala SAUERKRAUT, YOGURT, KOUMISS, FERMENTED CHEESE, APPLE CIDER VINEGAR, ACIDOPHILOUS and so on) that contains them. (see Insite# 39).

REVOLUTIONARY HEALTH INSITE #49: **PREPARED properly-- Meat is as BENEFICIAL as FRUITS & VEGETABLES (if not MORE SO)! And contains just as many ANTIOXIDANTS that EXTEND LIFESPAN!** In fact, certain ANTIOXIDANTS and INTRINSIC FACTORS that your Body absolutely MUST HAVE can ONLY come from MEAT! (such as CARNOSINE, URIC ACID, MYOGLOBIN and SATURATED FAT).

The PUSH by many RAW FOODISTS/VEGANS to stop the consumption of meat is a concerted effort that will just STARVE people in the midst of plenty!! (See BEHOLD THE PALE HORSE by Williams Cooper). Indeed—the VEGAN/RAW FOOD DIET is a STARVATION DIET!(one that should have DIED with the 60s as it grew more out of WHITE AMERIKAs Rebellious PROTEST against the VIETNAM WAR/CORPORATE GREED than a desire to HEAL bodies....now BLACK people have picked it up and are ILLING and KILLING themselves with this Diet)! If you are a BLACK VEGAN Man or Woman, put this book down rite now and RUN out and EAT you some GRASSFED BEEF!!!!

You are DYING from the inside out and dont even realize it! If you were meant to be totally HERBIVOROUS, your DIGESTIVE TRACT would be as long as any other Herbivorous Animal – or – you would have 3-4 stomachs like a COW!

However, if you insist on being a PLANT EATER then thatz ALL you should be eating. Otherwise, quit calling yourself a VEGAN anyway. Eating NUTS, SEEDS, GRAINS is NOT a True VEGAN. Thatz an OMNIVOROUS being—CALLING themselves VEGAN. Still, you are going to fool around and become MALNOURISHED even on THAT diet! I REPEAT: most of yawl NEED. MUST HAVE.

GOT TO HAVE. BETTER GET. Better EAT. Some MEAT! Before you DIE of MALNUTRITION! (see Insite# 0).

REVOLUTIONARY HEALTH INSITE #50: **The Standard ACID-ALKALINE Theory is not totally TRUE! Some People are SUPPOSED to be more ACID; while others are supposed to be more ALKALINE based on ETHNICITY!** BLACK/COLORED PEOPLE=more ACID. WHITE PEOPLE=more ALKALINE. This is why on average the WHITE BLOODSTREAM contains more WHITE BLOOD CELLS than those of the BLACK/COLORED ETHNICITIES. Thus, the food of the BLACK MAN/WOMAN should be more on the ACIDIC side as this matches the RESONANCE of Black BLOOD (its why we like more SALT, even SUGAR with our Foods....while those of the EUROCENTRIC ethnicity favor more BLAND foods—this is ALKALINE).

REVOLUTIONARY HEALTH INSITE #51: **You can NOT get all the PROTEIN, VITAMINS or MINERALS you need from VEGETABLES and/or PLANT foods!** Hell, you caint get all the PROTEIN you need from MEAT. So i know you can not get all the ones you need just from VEGETABLES and FRUIT! And please dont use the GORILLA or ELEPHANT example. You are neither one. Also it may help that both of them eat their Own SHIT! (Maybe thatz where the Real PROTEIN PAYOFF is....good lawd)! And another thing you may have overlooked about those two: they are A-N-I-M-A-L-S!! ANIMALS. A whole 'nother PHYSIOLOGY than YOURS. I guarantee you that if you tried to survive off of what a GORILLA ate--you would go APE!

REVOLUTIONARY HEALTH INSITE #52: **Make your own ELECTROLYTE Drink!** By mixing SUCANAT (nutritive sugar) and SEA SALT and/or BAKING SODA (non-aluminum). Half TEASPOON of both in 8 ounces of WARM water. Restores/Replaces the 4 major CELL SALTS, ie., CALCIUM, MAGNESIUM, POTASSIUM and SODIUM. The BODYs water content is mostly that of SEA SALT water anyway. SALINE-like. Just what you want. Your LYMPHATIC SYSTEM which is the primary benefactor of this treatment will Thank You because it controls your IMMUNE (defense) SYSTEM proper.

REVOLUTIONARY HEALTH INSITE #53: **Everybody has HERPES naturally in their body!**

So can we please STOP trying everything under the SUN to get rid of it! (getting in the SUN will help if you have a BREAK OUT tho). The HUMAN is born with the HERPES VIRUS as well as other Viruses as a Natural antidote. The ACTIVATION of the Herpes Virus (or any virus) comes about only when the body becomes to TOXIC (which weakens the IMMUNE SYSTEM) and becomes EXPOSED to the MATE of the particular OFFENDING virus*(often found in WHEAT and/or other GRAINS)!!* In other words, UNSANITARY conditions inside your body at time of the EXPOSURE to the MATING virus will ACTIVATE the DORMANT Herpes Virus (or other Corresponding virus). *This includes MRSA and other STAPHYLOCCOCUS Bacteria too that have a natural existence on the SKIN and in the NOSE.* Furthermore, having HERPES is a mutagenic protection whose vital properties actually enhance your immune system from other deadly viruses by protecting the cells! (The virus protects the cells that it moves into). (See the movie, INVASION with Nicole Kidman).

REVOLUTIONARY HEALTH INSITE #54:

DEPRESSION/SCHIZOPHRENIA can be CURED with LECITHIN and LITHIUM (aka The DOUBLE L DOSE)! *(see Insite #30).* LECITHIN OIL/FAT is said to make up ONE-THIRD of the BRAIN by Dry Weight; thus, its very crucial to the GOINGS-ON in the Brain. It is a precursor to many of the most important Khemicals that influence MENTAL STABILITY pathways, ie., SEROTONIN, MELATONIN, DOPAMINE, BETA ENDORPHINS, ENKEPHALINS, DYSNORPHINS—and as such affects, likewise the PINEAL and PITUITARY GLANDS, especially. This also means the LUTEINIZING HORMONES, PROGESTERONE, ESTROGEN, TESTOSTERONE hormones are affected too. Well, LECITHIN is involved in the making of them. Throw in CHOLESTEROL and CELL MEMBRANE integrity and you have yet 2 more critical reasons why one MUST have Lecithin! In fact, what I call the DOUBLE L DOSE<Lecithin and LITHIUM> are 2 of the MUST HAVE nutrients in trying to restore someone to MENTAL STABILITY. And must be kept in the EATIQUETTE (diet) for optimum Mental Clarity. Indeed, the WHOLE of the NERVOUS SYSTEM (think MYELIN SHEATHS, for example) ABSOLUTELY NEED the benefit of LECITHIN! Get Lecithin from: EGGS, CHEESE, Dairy products in general, LECITHIN OIL, NON-GMO SOYBEANS, PEANUTS, LIVER, HEART, TESTICLES, OVARIES, TRIPE (cow stomach), FISH FAT (omegas). Additionally, too low Cholesterol promotes SUICIDE in people who do not have sufficient amounts in their body. In fact, SUICIDES increase every WINTER. Why? 2 critical reasons that affect the body BIOKHEMICALLY: NO or LESS SUNLITE influences LOW SEROTONIN and LOW CHOLESTEROL.

Meanwhile, LITHIUM lines the Nerves of the NERVOUS SYSTEM as well, affecting

NEUTROTRANSMITTERS/RECEPTORS—which are damaged by DIETS high in URIC ACID caused by the consumption of too many REFINED CARBOHYDRATES and SUGAR which in turn exhausts your LITHIUM stores and raises the level of URIC ACID in the Blood. This results in MANIA, even PSYCHOSIS from the Lithium deficiency. Also results in TREMORS, SHAKES (Parkinsons, for example can be linked to LOW lithium). Get LITHIUM from LEMONS, LIMES, DARK GREEN VEGETABLES, NUTS, SEEDS, BEE POLLEN, ONIONS, TOMATOES, BAKING SODA (non-aluminum), SEAWEED, KELP, SEAMOSS, NATURAL MINERAL WATER.

REVOLUTIONARY HEALTH INSITE #55: **Building a FANTASTIC FETUS!** Call it BIRTH CONTROL of a (different) GOD kind. Indeed. A WOMAN can determine the quality of CHILD she will have based on what she EATS (or what she does NOT eat). The FRANKENMEDS call it FETAL PROGRAMMING.

The KEY is Your DIET in particular TRIMESTERS of pregnancy AFFECTs your BABY greatly! Meaning that during each TRIMESTER you need to make sure to EAT/DRINK certain NUTRIENTS to take advantage of that particular PHASE of FETAL GROWTH!! For example, LESS sugar in the FIRST trimester; Yet, more OIL. This is how we build GODS from the GROUND (ADAM/EVE) up! (and I doubt many of these HOSPITALS and INNERCITY CLINICS are trying to help women accomplish that)!!

Later adult episodes of DIABETES, HEART ATTACKS, OBESITY and/or BRAIN INTELLIGENCE are all determined by the NUTRIENTS taken during PREGNANCY. In short, if you want to give BIRTH to a GOD—you have to EAT like one while you are pregnant!

Of course, FETAL PROGRAMMING is not all that New. The IDEA has been around for a long time (after all, EUGENICS, which simply means GOOD GENES, is linked to FETAL PROGRAMMING when you think about it). However, its REBIRTH should not be lost on what this means to EXPECTANT mamas-to-be.

EAT RITE FOR YOUR CHILD TYPE: 6 of the Most IMPORTANT NUTRIENTS During PREGNANCY:
WATER, FAT (esp. OMEGA 3s and LECITHIN), B-VITAMINS (esp. FOLIC ACID, B-12, B-6, THIAMINE, NIACIN), LITHIUM (in the

form of SEA SALT), IRON, VITAMIN K, SELENIUM, CHLOROPHYLL, ZINC, SUN.

REVOLUTIONARY HEALTH INSITE #56: **Lack of PENIS HARDNESS is caused by CLOGGED ARTERIES!** A basic CIRCULATION issue. You have been EATING too much cooked/heated FAT which erodes/smothers the ARTERIES leading to the PENIS (or PEN-i for you smaller brothas)! And keeps it from SWELLING properly. You can help yourself a LOT by FASTING, MASSAGING (including TESTICLES, PERINEUM) and increased WATER intake w/moderate SEA SALT (1/4 teaspoon to a 8 oz. glass). Half-your-weight in OUNCES of Water overall. After a few weeks, start taking 2 tablespoons of RAW OIL (with and without FOOD), 2WICE a week. Also exercises that work the VAGUS NERVE (in the LUMBAR/base of the spine) will help.

REVOLUTIONARY HEALTH INSITE #57: **Women who can not ORGASM need to check their VAGUS NERVE function.** Blockages in the SOLAR PLEXUS and the NERVES leading up from the BASE of the SPINE can go offline due to EMOTIONAL trauma. 2 things: Heal the Emotions and EXERCISE the SPINE with proper MASSAGE and STRETCHING so that you target your VAGUS NERVE (Lumbar/Base Spine region). The Vagus Nerve serves as a sort of ON/OFF switch to ORGASMIC release! And it connects directly to the CLITORIS and the PINEAL GLAND. This Nerve which serves a capacitory job as a kinda Nerve Muscle, if you will, can HARDEN (atrophy) due to Dysfunctional LIFESTYLE inclusive of EMOTIONAL TRAUMA/SHOCK, DRUGS, improper SEXUAL HABITS and of course, DIET. It has to be REAWAKENED with a SERIOUS PHYSICAL and EMOTIONAL type of exercise. YOGA, PILATES, BIKRAM YOGA can all target this nerve. Even plain, old GYMNASTIC STRETCHING can help with this.

REVOLUTIONARY HEALTH INSITE #58: **STRETCHING is the Most Effective Exercise for the MUSCLE GROWTH (not just ELASTICITY)!** They are indeed FED by WORK (pushups, light weights, for example); but THRIVE and SURVIVE off of STRETCHING so that MELANIN (Myoglobin Pigments) move better thru the smaller muscles inside the muscles. Additionally, ACIDS can be circulated out of the MUSCLES as well. Stretching also takes PRESSURE off the NERVES that help the muscles fire efficiently.

REVOLUTIONARY HEALTH INSITE #59: **MENSTRUAL CRAMPS can be Cured by a DIET extremely HIGH in BIO-AVAILABLE foods!** CELL SALTS, FRUITS, VEGETABLES, WATER. CELL SALTS are (CALCIUM, MAGNESIUM, POTASSIUM and SODIUM, in other words ELECTROLYTES). A warm drink of say, SEA SALT, SUGAR (in the form of SUCANAT) is a great ELIXIR and helps with ELECTROLYTE Balance. Keep that in your EATING REGIMEN on a regular basis and you will have less problems from CRAMPS (provided you keep the FRUITS and VEGS at high level as well).

REVOLUTIONARY HEALTH INSITE #60: **Women give BIRTH to WATER BABIES!** Give your Child WATER as soon as you can in order to help them develop a taste for NATURAL FOODS. Your BABY has 20,000,000,000 billion CELLS! And everyone of them NEEDS Water!!(which is the Highest VIBRATORY FOOD for any MAN, WOMAN or CHILD). I know you hear that a baby should not drink Water (or that MUCH water)--but your BABY needs water. S/He is THIRSTY from the MOMENT they arrive here. And yes, your BREASTMILK is MOSTLY water----BUT that is NOT enough! It also contains SUGAR and SODIUM----which makes your Baby THIRSTY---thus, the child needs MORE water! Not much, you see. Just an additional 1-2 TABLESPOONS per BREASTFEEDING session. Give it to your BABY about 10 minutes AFTER she comes off the BREAST: 1 TABLESPOON of DISTILLED water would be great! Thatz NOT much. But its enough to help DIGEST breastmilk properly (which is full of MILKFAT, by the way). Babies need WATER too!

REVOLUTIONARY HEALTH INSITE #61: **ASTHMA is an ALLERGY due to FERMENTATION from SUGAR; which often affects small AIR SACS in the lungs.** SOULution? More water (half weight in ounces), oil (1-2 teaspoons coconut oil twice/week). High Sugar can attract mold, also known as pollen more intensely when the POLLEN COUNT is higher usual.

REVOLUTIONARY HEALTH INSITE #62: **BLACK PEOPLE (and people of color) do not have the same amount of WHITE BLOOD CELLS (on average) as White People.** This is important to know in terms of DIAGNOSING for Health Issues such as LUPUS where we can wind up being given DRUGS for a Disease that does not exist. And remember, the WBC Count (or even the RBC Count for that matter) is JUST A RANGE. Nothing else. If you are otherwise fine – do not sweat it. The COUNT you wanna be concerned about is your T-CELL COUNT. When that starts getting low – Then, there is cause for a little bit more concern. But your walking around everyday WBCs die off all the time. So that at any given time, they could be LOW or HIGHER. Depends on what is going on in your body or if you just ATE, CAUGHT the flue or whatever! WBCs are FINICKY. At any rate, keep your ZINC, B-COMPLEX, IODINE, CHLOROPILL stores up – and you will be okay overall.

REVOLUTIONARY HEALTH INSITE #63: **FOLLOW YOUR TEETH to Know WHAT to EAT!**

32 Teeth=Eating as opposed to ONLY drinking
20 MOLARS (fruits, vegetables, nuts and seeds);
8 INCISORS + 4 CANINES (meat, dairy, cheese, eggs)
Thus, 60% of your EATIQUETTE is for FRUITS, VEGETABLES, NUTS & SEEDS; and 40% for MEAT and Meat-BY PRODUCTS (DAIRY, EGGS, CHEESE)=100% eating. This can waiver between 80-20 as well.

REVOLUTIONARY HEALTH INSITE #64: **Drink HOT WATER!**

1--Balances ACID to ALKALINE ratio.

2--HARMONIZES CELLS to move in SYNCHRONY.

3--Is like drinking the SUN!

4--Helps VITAMIN D (especially, VITAMIN D3 and CALCIUM be released into the BLOODSTREAM properly).

REVOLUTIONARY HEALTH INSITE #65: **The VEGANISM and RAW FOODS MOVEMENT has DESTROYED just as many DIGESTIVE TRACTS as any other DISEASE over the last 40 years!** Why? Because it fails to understand that the VEGAN/RAW FOODS DIET is only for a CERTAIN period of time—that includes HEALING. To stay on it any longer than necessary brings on the OPPOSITE effect and it is NO LONGER Healing—rather it becomes one of continued SICKNESS—even DEATH to the individual as the body becomes DEFICIENT in Critical NUTRIENTS. VEGANISM, FRUITARIANISM and other MONO DIETS are NOT the ANSWER! Rather we must eat in a BALANCED manner from ALL of the FOOD GROUPS including MEAT and GRAINS (*however, not the normal ones instead BEANS/LEGUMES are the better Grains if we are to eat something called Grains).* This is a critical difference for it must be understood that any time in history where TRADITIONAL GRAINS have been introduced there has been SICKNESS and DECREASE in Lifespan! (Including KEMET/EGYPT)!

REVOLUTIONARY HEALTH INSITE #66: **WEIGHT GAIN/MAINTAIN Formula!**

You have STOPPED eating MEAT. But you are worried about LOSING too much WEIGHT and/or MAINTAINING your weight. What follows is a great TRANSITION formula that will help you adjust to life without MEAT. Here is what you do:

Buy the FOLLOWING items:

COCONUT (jelly-ish kind)

BANANAS

Virgin COCONUT oil

Virgin OLIVE oil

LECITHIN oil

EGGS (yes, Eggs....it is NOT like eating meat but IS meat).

WATER (DISTILLED----or boil it and POUR some non-aluminum baking soda or apple cider vinegar in it).

Next you want to BLEND:

1. COCONUT MEAT (healthy amount)
2. 2 BANANAS
3. 2-4 tablespoons of Coconut oil
4. 2-4 tablespoons of Olive oil
5. Half a teaspoon of LECITHIN
6. 1-ounce of distilled WATER
7. 1-2 SCRAMBLED eggs.
8. BLEND thoroughly.
9. Drink this 1-2 times per week.

...and your WEIGHT will MAINTAIN. If you are more interested in WEIGHT GAIN then you need to combine with WEIGHT

LIFTING, EXERCISE (meaning old-fashioned PUSHUPS, PULLUPS, SITUPS and so on) and STRETCHING.

REVOLUTIONARY HEALTH INSITE #67: **FASTING Builds and/or helps you Gain MUSCLE!!** This is due to its CLEANSING effect. MUSCLE TISSUE can get overloaded with TOXINS as well as any other organs (yes, they are ORGANS). FASTING clears this POLLUTION out which helps with OXYGENATION leading to more MYOGLOBIN (a Protein) in the Muscles to be expressed more efficiently; as well allowing better Muscle expansion and when combined with RESISTANCE WORK (not necessarily WEIGHTS—rather your own BODY WEIGHT in MOVEMENTS such as PUSHUPS, SITUPS, PULLUPS, LEG SQUATS). Plus, the increase in MYOGLOBIN PIGMENT helps with GLUCOSE into the Muscles without the help of Synthetic PROTEIN POWDERS/SUGARS—and this allows for SIZE and MASSIVENESS! Bodybuilders make the mistake of PROTEIN LOADING with SUGAR from PROTEIN POWDERS and Pure SUGAR rather than allowing the MUSCLES to FEED themselves with its own STORED Sugar—"and" FAT! The real growth comes from FAT not SUGAR per se (although it helps the process....*see Insite #73).*

REVOLUTIONARY HEALTH INSITE #68: **Every VITAMIN is a MULTIPLE VITAMIN!** Because it has MULTIPLE FUNCTIONS. And The best way to get these vitamins, however, is NOT thru SYNTHETIC VITAMINS in a BOTTLE—but thru your FOOD (as much as possible). At any rate, take VITAMIN B, for example: It has 17 STRAINS aka FUNCTIONS---Vitamin D has at least 3 (but there are more that simply have not been discovered--and thus go UN-NAMED)-- Vitamin K has at least 2 STRAINS. Again there are more. Said another way: every VITAMIN has MULTIPLE FUNCTIONS inside the BODY proper. And when you FAST, you encourage the body to RELEASE its Vitamin/Mineral contents in order to REGENERATE its ORGANS. (see Insite #164)

REVOLUTIONARY HEALTH INSITE #69: **Every Khemical in WEED that gives you ENLIGHTENMENT—you have it ALREADY inside your Brain!! Therefore, WEED should NOT be SMOKED (TOKED) without the Supervision of a respected elder who knows the REAL properties of the Drug. For Weed is basically a MEDICINE that should only be used for SACRED, RITUALISTIC, HEALING, purposes by a RESPONSIBLE being.** Otherwise, its use tends to result in RECREATIONAL smoking that accomplishes NOTHING but Laziness. (although at first, it may seem like you have found the MOST HIGH—when its really just being the MOST HIGH....lol)!

Furthermore, WEED affects critical BRAIN RECEPTORS that control SANITY and THINKING, both of which can be destroyed over time from constant taking of it. Learn to MEDITATE instead of WEEDITATE! For MEDITATION accomplishes ALL of the SAME goals of Weed WITHOUT the SIDE EFFECTS. And its LEGAL and you can do it anywhere! This is what the ANCIENTS showed us thru their efforts. That you can RAISE your level of VIBRATION by ALTERING your OWN mind with the Natural ENDOGENOUS (inside) CANNIBOIDS in your BRAIN!! (sitting in the HYPOTHALAMUS, PITUITARY, PINEAL GLANDS, NERVOUS SYSTEM proper--even the REPRODUCTIVE SYSTEM which is one reason you get Mad Libido).

The additional problem with WEED is that many people have a high level of *THC RECEPTORS* which matches with that of weed—and this BLOWS a FUSE! Resulting in your getting a DOUBLE DOSE of the GREENY GREEN! Its too much and with constant use your BRAIN MATTER begins to develop small, PINPRICK-like size holes (thatz NOT A GOOD LOOK)! And you will begin to lose your ability to REASON. And well you should because this is a reflection of DOPAMINE which steals reasoning from the FRONTAL LOBE (forebrain).

REVOLUTIONARY HEALTH INSITE #70: **DEPRESSION as well as any other MENTAL ILLNESS (Suicidal Thoughts, Alzheimers, Anorexia, Bulimia and so on) can be CURED by Staying AWAKE!** In other words, Do NOT go to BED. This form of SLEEP DEPRIVATION keeps high levels of BRAIN NEUROGENESIS DERIVED FACTOR, a Nervous System Hormone that helps your Brain build more NEW nerve cells and keeps your Brain growing with new Neuronal Connections; this in turn contributes to SEROTONIN and DOPAMINE circulating in your BRAIN. And both of these Natural Khemicals are MOOD ENHANCERS for the Better! They keep you HAPPY and SHARP! Do it in PHASES. If you get up at 12midnite, you stay up til the NEXT midnite—and then go to bed sometime after that. When you wake up, IMMEDIATELY go and STARE into a BRIGHT LITE or the SUN whichever. This helps maintain your CHEMICAL BALANCE of SEROTONIN, BETA ENDORPPHINS and other Brain juices that are critical to keeping you MENTALLY STABLE. Also start increasing your intake of FATTY OILS (Butter, virgin Coconut Oil, for example), also EXERCISE (to keep BLOOD circulating with OXYGEN to the Brain), as well as Eat more PROTEIN (helps STIMULATE endogenous <inside> GLUTAMATE and GABA which are additional NEURO/BRAIN TRANSMITTERS in the Brain proper). Invest in a UVB LITE if you can which will help produce MELATONIN and PIGMENT at the CELLULAR level as well. *(see Insite #54).*

REVOLUTIONARY HEALTH INSITE #71: **X-RAYS are HARMLESS! (overall).** Do not trip on the X-RAY. Itz not enuff RADIATION to hurt the BODY. So do NOT be scared of that. The X-RAY production is just to IMPRESS you. Putting on a STEEL JACKET they have. The big lites. Kool looking equipment. Itz smoke and mirrors! There is not enuff Radiation coming out of the thing to hurt you. Otherwise, you would have on a PROTECTIVE VEST too! How many people do you know that have died from X-RAY exposure/exams? Now, X-RADIATION! thatz a different thing my people!! However, the level of light they use for X-RAYS is among the most HARMLESS LIGHTS in the SPECTRUM. It is basically WHITE LIGHT (like from the average 60 watt bulb!)--and BLUE/BLACK/PURPLE LIGHT forming a prism by mixing. Both relatively HARMLESS! And thatz all an X-RAY is. Throw in a little GAS and you got it. If anything was going to kill you it would be the GAS. But there aint enuff of it in X-RAY LITE, either. There is in a NUCLEAR REACTOR. an ATOM BOMB too. But not an X-RAY.

REVOLUTIONARY HEALTH INSITE #72: **BLOOD actually has more of a NEUTRAL PH (like WATER); while it is the LYMPH that has more of a RANGE in PH!** (something generally CREDITED to the BLOOD). It is the LYMPH tissue that is the one that must be kept at a level PH BALANCE. How do we know? Because it is the LYMPH that services the BLOOD. The Blood does NOT service the LYMPH. It is the LYMPH that carries the WHITE BLOOD CELLS' TRASH when the WBCs CLEAN and MOP up. Thus, BLOOD is the one that is most NEUTRAL at about 7.0 PH. The LYMPH goes from 3.0 (death—CONCENTRATED ACID) to 12 (death—DILUTED ACID). But is generally in the range of 7.0 to 7.4. The only way the BLOOD does not remain neutral is if the LYMPH is BROKEN DOWN and the WBCs get into the BLOODSTREAM in an attempt to clean up. Then, the Blood becomes more CONCENTRATED ACID.

REVOLUTIONARY HEALTH INSITE #73: **PROTEIN is Not the MUSCLE BUILDER!** Yeah, its in the MUSCLES—but its not what BUILDS the muscles. Its ESSENTIAL for the muscles. But its not what BUILDS the Muscles. If your body is not showing signs of MUSCLE-WASTING I would NOT worry about PROTEIN DEFICIENCY. The muscles use Proteins, of course. Even stores it. But you do not BUILD more MUSCLE on more PROTEIN in a normally healthy body. A SICK, WASTING body. Yes! That body needs more PROTEIN because it is losing protein out of the muscles. Most of us are not. (Altho some of you experiencing FIBROMYALGIA may be losing protein, like a protein leak...get your PROTEIN LEVELS checked if you are experiencing Fibromyalgia...and NOT just the KIDNEYS only, get the LIVER examined, too, for that protein leak as well...The LIVER stores proteins/vitamins/minerals...yet the KIDNEY is always checked for protein loss via the URINE. Thatz gonna give you a FALSE POSITIVE reading. It may or may not show up. Do both really).

Anyway, PROTEIN is NOT what makes MUSCLE grow!! It helps. True. But Itz really WATER, FAT and SUGAR (GLUCOSES of which there are 8 main ones) SYNTHESIS that brings on the Muscle growth! Bodybuilders/Strongmen are chasing Protein when they need to be chasing WATER, FAT and SUGAR!! Your body can ONLY hold about 1% worth of protein at one time. You can not eat more EVERYDAY and expect that protein to be assimilated. It WILL NOT be! It is STORED instead. Big difference. Therefore, any MUSCLE GROWTH that you have is NOT the result of PROTEIN ASSIMILATION but of WATER, FAT and SUGAR synthesis. *(see Insite #67).*

REVOLUTIONARY HEALTH INSITE #74: **PEEL your TOOTH and GUM DECAY Away!** With Citrus. Rub the inside of a LEMON/LIME/GRAPEFRUIT peel on your GUMS. Simply massage the peel in and around your gums. Get the entire mouth. Make sure the PEEL still has a little FRUIT MEAT (fiber) left inside it. VITAMIN C is QUEEN when it comes to HEALING up CONNECTIVE TISSUE. And thatz what your GUMS are: CONNECTIVE, ELASTIC TISSUE. A LEMON JUICE rinse is good too. Just RINSE your mouth out 60 seconds later with distilled water. Also swallowing the LEMON JUICE increases your BONE DENSITY levels (as you well know VITAMIN C helps with SCURVY and thus ELASTIC TISSUE & BONES). NUTS/SEEDS are your best bet for the CALCIUM (and PHOSPHOROUS). For example, SESAME seeds. ALMONDS (the sliced, blanched ones...the whole Almonds are for a different healing remedy). Combining the CITRUS PEEL MASSAGE, getting more VITAMIN C in your eating (either via FRUITS or a liquid vite C) and organic CALCIUM will help your TEETH out a lot. Because Vitamin C and Calcium are two the most important elements to our TEETH as we age from 12-13 on up.

REVOLUTIONARY HEALTH INSITE # 75: **Having SEX during PREGNANCY creates a much needed CONNECTION between the BABY and FATHER! Because during the ACT the Father releases TESTOSTERONE via his SPERM which confers further IMMUNITY to the embryo!** And if you are a father and you know your sperm is healthy as hell—you should be releasing it as much as possible so that it finds its way into the PLACENTA with the baby. S/He needs that. This is additionally needed because LACK of Testosterone is one of the main REASONS that many children are born with PHYSICAL DEFORMITIES (can not grow, no coordination). That Testosterone is an ANABOLIC STEROID that promotes MUSCLE and PUBERTY in the correct amount. If it is DEFICIENT in UTERO it can affect the child just as well as too little ESTROGEN (or too much). *NOTE: Testosterone is NOT the only thing that makes for Physical deformities, of course.* Just remember to go easy with the THRUSTING, fellas!

REVOLUTIONARY HEALTH INSITE #76: **WALK if you want the easiest PREGNANCY DELIVERY possible!** And don't stop walking all of your PREGNANCY. Rite up until you bout to have that BABY---be walking! That baby will damn near just FALL rite out of you with a FEW pushes!

REVOLUTIONARY HEALTH INSITE #77: **There are SUN FOODS and MOON FOODS that we must eat to be in HARMONY with the SUPER FORCES of this world!** FRUITS in the DAY; VEGETABLES at NITE. Or said another way: LEMONS, LIMES, ORANGES, BERRIES and so on in the DAYTIME. And TOMATOES, ONIONS, PEPPERS, SPICES in the NITETIME.

REVOLUTIONARY HEALTH INSITE #78: **The SABBATH DAY for you is your BIRTHDAY!** Therefore, FAST/REST/MEDITATE for long periods of time on this day.

REVOLUTIONARY HEALTH INSITE #79: **You need never SUPPLEMENT since All the NUTRIENTS that you will ever need are ALREADY inside your CELLS!** Waiting to be ACTIVATED by PROPER nutrients from FOOD or other ALTERNATIVE or UNEXPECTED SOURCES such as SUNLITE, MOONLITE, GOOD AIR and DISTILLED WATER....this is a main reason it is important to have a CORRECT Eating Regimen, combined with the proper ENVIRONMENT/GEOGRAPHICAL LOCATION and frame of MIND. Yes, there can be exceptions to this SUPPLEMENTATIN RULE (extreme sickness/illness, rehab, recovery, really bad pollution, extremely bad eating or unhealthy lifestyles and so on)

REVOLUTIONARY HEALTH INSITE #80: **STOP EATING for 24-48 hours every 10-12 days.** For the ENTIRE 24-48 hours! DON'T EAT A DAMN THANG! NOTHING. ZERO! This will TRULY take a LOAD off your----ORGANS! Allowing them to rest, detoxify and regenerate their cells.

REVOLUTIONARY HEALTH INSITE #81: **The CURE for a Weak heart is OIL and WATER!** (yup, they do MIX, at least in this equation). The THICKER the oil, the Better (ala FLAXSEED, CODLIVER or LECITHIN, even SESAME SEED can be used). Hit that oil 'bout 2wice a month/1-2 ounces each time (depending on how WEAK your heart is; an EKG will tell you that.

REVOLUTIONARY HEALTH INSITE #82: **2 OUNCES of oil is EQUAL to 16 ounces of WATER!** And we must therefore drink as much OIL, relatively speaking, as we do WATER (at least once every 2 weeks or more depending on how DEFICIENT you are). As a people, we are not only DEHYDRATED but RUSTED! LOL! (think FIBROMYALGIA).

REVOLUTIONARY HEALTH INSITE #83: **A too-ALKALINE environment can be just as SICKENING as a too-ACID environment! An overproduction of either one be cause for DISEASE!** For example, MOST of your FLUS, COLDS, BACTERIAS, VIRUSES thrive in an ALKALINE (WINTER) environment inside the body. Whereas other Diseases like the MOLD that produces CANCER thrives in an ACID (SUMMER) environment inside the body. We are always hearing about being TOO Acid. Yet, you can also be TOO ALKALINE as well. Ironically, one of the best PREVENTIVE cures for COLDS is COLD AIR (even Cold Showers); while one of the best CURES for CANCER (preventive or otherwise)is the HEAT from the SUN!

REVOLUTIONARY HEALTH INSITE #84: **Its better to JUDGE food based on how it SMELLS rather than how it TASTES!** This is due to the TONGUE being subject to chemical manipulation; and easily TRAINED to love foods that the body can NOT use. However, SMELL is much older and reliable than all of the SENSES (maybe, with the exception of HEARING). You see, our TONGUES are connected to the TYMPANI NERVE which is part of one of the 12 (some say 13) CRANIAL nerves emerging from the BRAIN. And this is a TASTE RECEPTOR site that governs TASTE SENSATIONS----The problem with this is that this NERVE can be easily CORRUPTED by KHEMICALS (TOXINS, really)----or said another way: your TASTE can be ALTERED dramatically via this nerve! And you can/will fall in love with KHEMICALS themselves rather than the True pure, nature of the food. *(see Insite #143).*

REVOLUTIONARY HEALTH INSITE #85: **MALE EJACULATION or SQUIRTING (Female Ejaculation) Both DRAIN the ENDOCRINE SYSTEMS of the MAN or WOMAN--and should be reserved.** In fact, FEMALE EJACULATION while considered NORMAL by many SEXUAL ENTHUSIASTS (for its ORGASMIC POWER) is actually very Detrimental to the entire HORMONAL SYSTEM of the Woman-who LOSES a variety of vital minerals just like the man from what has now become a recreational sport of PORNO proportions! (in fact, it is the world of PORNOGRAPHY that has made this popular).

REVOLUTIONARY HEALTH INSITE #86: Use **WALNUT TEA for DEPRESSION.** Why? Walnuts produce the BRAIN KHEMICAL called SEROTONIN which is the HAPPINESS dope inside the Brain (which manufactures over 40 different types of NATURAL drugs, ie., SEROTONIN, DOPAMINE, MELATONIN, TRYPTOPHAN). Of course, its no surprise that the Walnut is even SHAPED like the BRAIN relating to the DOCTRINE OF SIGNATURES (=that which a fruit, vegetable, herb is shaped like is the part of the body it Heals).

REVOLUTIONARY HEALTH INSITE #87: **The 4 GRAINS to AVOID: RYE, WHEAT, BARLEY & WHITE BREAD!** Our BIOSYSTEMS can NOT handle the GLUTEN contained in these so-called particular foods. In 10,000 years of Eating them, our bodies STILL have not adjusted to MOST grains! (mainly, because they are not meant for human consumption). Thus, we suffer AUTOIMMUNE DISEASES (lupus, fibromyalgia, sickle cell, anemia and multiple sclerosis to name a few).

REVOLUTIONARY HEALTH INSITE #88: **The Highest levels of CHOLESTEROL are found in the LONGEST LIVED peeples!** Why? Because contrary to the SELF-INTERESTS of the MEDICAL MAFIA the CHOLESTEROL, in your BLOOD is a PROTECTIVE mechanism--more than a HARMFUL one. Furthermore, there is no GOOD or BAD cholesterol. Only a Good or Bad DIET.

REVOLUTIONARY HEALTH INSITE #89: **EMOTIONS Cause DIS-EASE.** And in fact, Emotions are attached to EVERY Disease the HUMAN Plant is afflicted with. Therefore, one must not only HEAL the SYMPTOM (disease), but also Heal the UNDERLYING Emotion. Only then can we say there has been a TRUE Healing.

REVOLUTIONARY HEALTH INSITE #90: **One of the greatest CURES for keeping your BLOODSTREAM in its correct PH BALANCE (Proper Homeostatic Balance) is POSITIVE THOUGHT PROCESSES** (which by itself can move your PH from 7.4+ down to 7.3 which is where BLOOD was before the 1800s)! Thus, combine good FOOD with good THOUGHTS for the good, long LIFE!

REVOLUTIONARY HEALTH INSITE #91: **EATING is Less a Source of ENERGY to the HUMAN BODY than we realize.** Actually, eating is a DRAIN on the ENERGY RESERVES of the body. This is why its CRITICAL that we learn how to maximize ALTERNATE energy PATHWAYS (ie., SUN, WATER, FASTING, DEEP BREATHING, EXERCISE, MEDITATION). Thus, our WRONG misconception about eating is what causes our tendency to OVEREAT to the point of SICKNESS and DISEASE!

REVOLUTIONARY HEALTH INSITE #92: **The Body needs OIL just as much as it Needs WATER!** In fact, to stay Well-Oiled one must consume at least 2-4 ounces of PURE oil every 10-12 days; while drinking at least 40-64 ounces of (distilled/alkaline) WATER daily or MORE depending on your SIZE. 2 ounces of OIL is equal to 32 ounces of (distilled) WATER. Virgin COCONUT OIL, BUTTER OIL, COD LIVER OIL or Extra Virgin OLIVE OIL are all good choices.

REVOLUTIONARY HEALTH INSITE #93: **If you are going to SUPPLEMENT with VITAMINS and MINERALS your BEST BET is to get your SUPPLEMENTATION from Individual (renegade) DOCTORS rather than COMPANIES**. And preferably, in Liquid or Powder form. However, we need to understand that, as a Rule, the body has ALL of the NUTRITITVE ELEMENTS it will ever need locked inside its CELLS. The MORE of LIVE, WHOLE FOODS that you eat, the MORE you will have NUTRIENTS available to your CELLS—and the LESS you have to worry about SUPPLEMENTING. Thus, stay away from REFINED CARBS/PROCESSED FOODS which deliver ABSOLUTELY NOTHING to your cells except DISEASE!

REVOLUTIONARY HEALTH INSITE #94: **You need to EAT/DRINK different OILS in different Seasons in order for your VEINS to remain in the best condition (you are only as OLD as your VEINS).** LIGHTER/THINNER/OMEGA-3, MONOSATURATED/SATURED oils (OLIVE, COCONUT, SUNFLOWER) in the SUMMER, HOTTER months; and HEAVIER/THICKER/SATURATED and OMEGA-6 type oils (Coconut which can be used for both seasons, CODLIVER, SESAME, BUTTER or HEMP oils) in the WINTER, COLDER months. The VEINS in the body require THINNESS or THICKNESS much like a car requires different Oil VISCOSITIES when the weather changes.

REVOLUTIONARY HEALTH INSITE #95: **We survive in 2 ways: DIRECT SUNLITE and DIRECT FOOD NUTRIENTS.** Our BLOOD CELLS are like SOLAR PANELS which extract ENERGY directly from the SUN so that we may live. Then, our SOMATIC CELLS (from the LIVER, KIDNEYS, BRAIN, HEART and so on), extract Energy directly from the FOODS we eat to keep our ORGANS working.

REVOLUTIONARY HEALTH INSITE #96: **The BEST time to increase (even double) your MELANIN stores in the SKIN as well as VITAMIN D content are the hours between 10am-2pm.** The SUN is at HER highest at this POINT and pregnant with UVB Rays (the safest ones of all for the HUMAN PLANT to absorb)."

REVOLUTIONARY HEALTH INSITE #97: **WEIGHTLIFTING (preferably, Your Own BODYWEIGHT, however use LIGHT WEIGHTS if you do use weights) is the single best way to RE-MINERALIZE the BONES of the body.** The PRESSURE forces all requisite CELLS (OSTEBLASTS, OSTEOCLASTS and OSTEOCYTES) to produce MORE bone matrix—and become DENSER, thicker. This principle can also be applied to Re-mineralizing your TEETH: thru CLINCHING (the Teeth together. This forces BONE (which the Teeth are a form of Bone) to grow. And by RINSING your mouth with (non-aluminum) BAKING SODA daily delivers CELL SALTS to the ENAMEL which feeds them.

REVOLUTIONARY HEALTH INSITE #98: **The 1/100th POINT DIFFERENCE** has many people in a condition known as the WALKING SICK. You are not bed-ridden, but you just never feel really good. Thats that 1/100th in effect. It means that you are most likely a little below where your PH BALANCE should be (averaging 7.35 - 7.4 depending on the individual). The question is WHY? The Why can/will determine the TREATMENT/CURE.

REVOLUTIONARY HEALTH INSITE #99: **Eat FRUITS in the day; SALADS and/or MEAT in the AFTERNOON; and ROOT VEGETABLES (sweet potatoes, carrots) in the EVENING** for the best BALANCING of your HORMONES.

REVOLUTIONARY HEALTH INSITE #100: **Use DEEP BREATHING instead of VIAGRA.** Better to MIMIC the EFFECTS of Viagra with LUNG MOVEMENT. Yes, it takes longer but it BUILDS up the WHOLE(listic) VASCULAR/CIRCULATORY system—as well as promotes HUMAN GROWTH HORMONES at a SAFE Dose the body can handle. Meanwhile, the VIAGRA Dose that Doctors prescribe is too high!! The body also benefits from additional OXYGEN-INDUCED Hormones including TESTOTERONE/ANDGROGEN (men); ESTROGEN,PROGESTERONE (women); and more production of RED BLOOD CELLS. Start your DEEP BREATHING efforts real easy. Build up to repeating the Deep Breaths many, many times! On the other hand, VIAGRA exhausts your VASCULAR (vein) system with steady use. Promoting High BLOOD PRESSURE, PENILE TISSUE DAMAGE, HEADACHES, SENILITY, and the list goes on. You will have a HARD PENIS at the risk of getting a SOFT (feeble) MIND.

REVOLUTIONARY HEALTH INSITE #101: MEDISIN **is focused on DISEASE rather than HEALTH;** On the CURE rather than PREVENTION; on PROFIT rather than PEOPLE; and on DEATH rather than LIFE. And they call this HEALING."

REVOLUTIONARY HEALTH INSITE #102: **The Best SUGAR for the HUMAN BODY is in SWEET & SOUR FRUITS** like POMEGRANATES, LEMONS, LIMES, GRAPEFRUITS, BERRIES, CHERRIES, GRAPES, ELDERBERRIES. These Fruits also contain adequate amounts of Natural SALT too.

REVOLUTIONARY HEALTH INSITE #103: **The Best SALT (Sodium) for the HUMAN BODY is in SOUR & SALT FRUIT/VEGETABLES** like TOMATOES, ONIONS, CUCUMBERS, LEMONS, LIMES, GRAPEFRUITS, SAUERKRAUT. These Vegetables also contain decent amount of Natural SUGAR as well.

REVOLUTIONARY HEALTH INSITE #104: **Despite what RAW FOODISTS and/or VEGANS say: COOKING does Not DESTROY the Life of REAL, LIVE, WHOLE Foods!** The NUTRIENTS in REAL foods can not be KILLED. Nutrients are ENERGY and Energy can not be DESTROYED. Therefore, HEAT will not HARM it. The HUMAN PLANT can consume both COOKED (Heat-Altered) and RAW foods as a path to Health. The Time-Honored Cultural practice of BOILING/STEWING/STEAMING is the best, safest way to HEAT/COOK your foods. And this will PRESERVE as well as PRE-DIGEST foods. That is to say, that certain foods like VEGETABLES (Broccoli, Tubers such as Sweet Potatoes); or MEATS "need" to be HEATED in order that the body can better ASSIMILATE/ABSORB their Nutrients. *(see my other book, The IMMORTALITY GUIDE).*

REVOLUTIONARY HEALTH INSITE #105: **CONSTIPATION is a little-known side effect of HORMONAL issues!** You see, CONSTIPATION is NOT just an a problem with simply EATING the wrong FOODS (altho that can figure in, of course); your HORMONES get their SIGNALS from the Mama GLAND of the Body: the HYPOTHALAMUS which in turn Controls the PITUITARY and signals it to produce HORMONES. The Hypothalamus ALSO signals THIRST and BOWEL MOVEMENTS--thus, if one has a problem with CONSTIPATION and/or HORMONES--it involves the SAME Gland which controls them both. They often go HAND-IN-HAND. So its NOT uncommon to have Hormonal issues and suffer with Constipation too!

REVOLUTIONARY HEALTH INSITE #106: **The GENETIC THEORY of DIS-EASE is a LIE--because GENES are NOT the problem in Dis-ease.** Show me a GENETIC DEFORMITY and I will show you a NUTRITIONAL DEFICIENCY. Its not BAD Genes that are passed on--rather it is BAD NUTRITIONAL HABITS that are passed from PARENT to CHILD. It must be understood the GENE itself is but an ORGAN! And as such can be DEFORMED due to LACK rite NUTRIENTS.

REVOLUTIONARY HEALTH INSITE #107: **Make the NUTRIENTS in Your FOOD work for Your BODY rather than MAKING your Body work for the NUTRIENTS** (using up its own ORGANIC MATERIAL to manufacture Nutrients because the Foods you eat have none). Thus, concentrate on EATING those foods that ALWAYS Assimilate/Absorb the easiest (Fruits, Vegetables).

REVOLUTIONARY HEALTH INSITE #108: **It is just as easy to become a FOOD ADDICT from FOOD ADDITIVES as it is to become a DOPE ADDICT from DRUGS.** Our Foods of today are not FOODS at all rather they are ADDICTIVE SUBSTANCES masquerading as SUSTENANCE.

REVOLUTIONARY HEALTH INSITE #109: **A DIABETIC is the SAME as a DYING ADDICT!** Except the DRUG of Choice is INSULIN rather than HEROIN!

REVOLUTIONARY HEALTH INSITE #110: **KETOSIS is the Natural, Physiological state of the HUMAN BODY!** Ketosis, which is FAT BURNING, allows the body to run off its own FAT STORES rather than GLUCOSE as its fuel. This promotes a SLOW DOWN in AGING; while decreasing DISEASE conditions. We have been sold a LIE that tells us we MUST run off of CARBOHYDRATES for fuel. This allows INDUSTRY to market their EMPTY, REFINED carbohydrates to us that do nothing except make us SICK! GLUCOSE in the form of CARBS is the SECONDARY fuel of the body. Not the PRIMARY one as we are SOLD/TOLD to keep us eating like PIGS due to all the unnecessary INSULIN production/stimulation!

KETOSIS also allows your body to ACTIVATE its PARASYMPATHETIC NERVOUS SYSTEM which gives you time to Organs time to REST from STRESS. This is the same idea behind EASTERN MEDITATION—activating the Parasympathetic Nervous System. Additionally, you increase the use of GLUCAGON in the body rather than the constant use of GLUCOSE. Glucagon goes hand-in-hand with your PNS which lessens INSULIN and CORTSOL production both which are HORMONES that DRAINS the Batteries (ADRENALS) of the body! This leads to RAPID AGING from overuse of the SYMPATHETIC NERVOUS SYSTEMS where the ADRENALS live.

REVOLUTIONARY HEALTH INSITE #111: **SUGAR forces FAT (TRIGLYCERIDES) out of the LIVER!** And this Exhausts the PANCREAS too by making it produce too much INSULIN instead of GLUCAGON. We must understand that INSULIN is the STRESS Sugar; while GLUCAGON is the REST Sugar! Insulin production wears the body out as it partners with CORTISOL (an ADRENALINE HORMONE that truly TAXES the body when its NOT needed) via the SYMPATHETIC NERVOUS SYSTEM; on the other hand Glucagon CALMS the body as it uses more the PARASYMPATHETIC NERVOUS SYSTEM.

REVOLUTIONARY HEALTH INSITE #112: **It is Not DIS-EASE that is INCURABLE**, rather its a MEDICAL MAFIA that TELLS US that Dis-ease is INCURABLE.

REVOLUTIONARY HEALTH INSITE #113: T**here are ONLY 4 NUTRIENTS that really count in the Body: SALT, SUGAR, FAT or WATER!** The BASIC RECIPE of Life. All these other words, ie., Protein, Carbon, Minerals, Vitamins, Hormones, Sterols, Blood–are simply a COMPOSITION of these FOUR! (and they mostly CONFUSE the issue). These 4 ELEMENTS cover everything in the HUMAN PLANT (for indeed, we are PLANTS). Together they are the NUTRIENTS that keep us Alive.

REVOLUTIONARY HEALTH INSITE #114: T**o Heal the THYROID & neglect the THYMUS is a critical mistake.** Both these GLANDS are important to IMMNUNITY. Both NUTRIENTS were potent CATALYSTS in the START of LIFE itself from a MICROBACTERIA-laden, PROBIOTIC SOUP. When the THYMUS GLAND is missing Nutrients—BEHAVIOR changes from PEACE to WAR! The Thymus SHRINKS or ATROPHIES unless it is fed properly. The Thyroid needs IODINE; and the Thymus needs SELENIUM.

REVOLUTIONARY HEALTH INSITE #115: **AGING and DEATH are DISEASES that have been PROGRAMMED into the ROOT CONSCIOUSNESS of HUMAN SOCIETY**. Yet, they are MALADIES that can be ELIMINATED with the proper RE-SEEDING of Self.

REVOLUTIONARY HEALTH INSITE #116: C**ontrary to what the MAINSTREAM MEDIA is SELLING us: Americans actually have a DECLINING lifespan rather than an EXTENDED one.** Compared to how long we USED to live (and are SUPPOSED to live). A BIG reason for this number? ADRENAL EXHAUSTION via INSULIN/CORTISOL production due to STRESS, STRESS, STRESS and more STRESS—brought on by Bad foods and highly EMOTIONAL lifestyles.

REVOLUTIONARY HEALTH INSITE #117: **Maybe the reason so many People DIE in HOSPITALS** is because the HOSPITALS are Full of S.H.I.T. (STANDARD HEALTHCARE INDUSTRY TREATMENT)! For example, DOCTOR ERROR is (arguably) 3rd leading cause of DEATH. In fact, many of the INFECTIOUS DISEASES we suffer from in the general population—starts in the smaller populous of HOSPITAL STAFFS including most VIRAL Diseases such as TUBERCULOSIS, AIDS; and of course, one of the current favorites--MRSA!! For the most part, the way Hospitals are operated they are essentially INCUBATORS for giving people DISEASES—and CAUSING more of the same!

REVOLUTIONARY HEALTH INSITE #118: **A WATER and JUICE FAST, Alternating days (on/off like 2-4 days Fasting) for up to 60 days will CLEAN and DISSOLVE PARASITES out of the CECUM** which sits at the end of the COLON and is where most of PARASITES live inside your body. The CECUM is their home. They manufacture a chemical called CYTASE that is used for DISINFECTANT for any BACTERIA that gets out of control in the DIGESTIVE TRACT. This prevents the start of CANCER and/or other SEPTIC ILLNESSES.

REVOLUTIONARY HEALTH INSITE #119: **Not HEALTHCARE** rather HEALTHYSELF CARE!

REVOLUTIONARY HEALTH INSITE #120: **The WAR on DRUGS needs to include PRESCRIPTION DRUGS—and even some VITAMINS/MINERALS and other SUPPLEMENTS!** In fact, this IS the WAR in the final analysis because all the NATURAL drugs are used to MAKE these PRESCRIPTION drugs that the MEDICAL MAFIA wants to use to control our BRAINS.

REVOLUTIONARY HEALTH INSITE #121: **DRINK as much WATER in the WINTER as in the SUMMER. And Add IODIZED SEA SALT to the WATER. LACK of SALT contributes to many NERVE DISEASES (MS, PARKINSONS, ALZHEIMER).** Also INCREASE the amount of FATS/CHOLESTEROL (which guards against DEPRESSION/SEASONAL AFFECTATION DISORDER) as a protective mechanism for the BLOOD which needs to CHANGE to a THICKER weight.

REVOLUTIONARY HEALTH INSITE #122: **We must increasingly understand what I call ANCESTRAL HEALING EATIQUETTE**--which tells us HOW you must eat; WHAT you must eat; WHEN you must eat; WHY you must eat What you eat; based on the PEOPLE of your Lineage WHO ate like you before; and WHERE they ate when they were eating. Only then, can a PROPER of EATING (aka EATIQUETTE) be established for You.

REVOLUTIONARY HEALTH INSITE #123: **You are not SICK, your BODY** is just trying to TELL you SOMETHING!

REVOLUTIONARY HEALTH INSITE #124: **You can no more EAT the SAME DIET as someone else as you can have the Same FINGERPRINT or DNA.** You are UNIQUE! Your METABOLISM is a reflection of YOUR "particular" Molecular Structure." Thus, RAW FOODISM, FRUITARIANSIM, VEGANISM or VEGETARIANISM is NOT for everyone despite those who say it is. You have to EAT FOR YOU not your BOO—or even BOO the FOO! And this may include eating MEAT!

REVOLUTIONARY HEALTH INSITE #125: **The DOKTOR of today is more like a Mad SCIENTIST than a True HEALER.** Their view of PEOPLE is more as GUINEA PIGS to be EXPERIMENTED upon than HEALED.

REVOLUTIONARY HEALTH INSITES #126: **As a Rule: GRAINS are not good for HUMAN consumption.** Even ANIMALS are not built for eating Grains! GRAINS kill them much earlier than their natural DIET of GRASS, PLANTS, VEGETABLES, FRUITS. Likewise, Grains are not meant for Human eating either. ANIMALS who eat Grains have many of the SAME health issues as HUMANS! (arthritis, mental illness, for example). Thus, it is Grains we need to avoid like the PLAGUE! They produce too many HEALTH problems. Additionally, Another point about GRAINS: They Force BLOOD GLUCOSE up too much! And the body caint handle that much SUGAR. Plus, too many POISONS (phytates) which make LECTINS causing the Blood to HEMAGLUTINNATE (clump). This then forces the body to make ANTIBODIES that have a hard time recognizing GRAIN PROTEINS (which then go on to wreck havoc on the tissues—causing infamous AUTOIMMUNE DISEASES like CELIAC, LUPUS, FIBROMYALGIA and DIABETES).

REVOLUTIONARY HEALTH INSITE #127: **FRUITS and VEGETABLES (to a lessa degree) are the most Powerful HERBS that we can actually take into our bodies for HEALTH!** All the so-called other traditional Herbs are more DRUGS than FOODS. And should be used as such.

REVOLUTIONARY HEALTH INSITE #128: **A True FOOD is MEDICINE; everything else is a DRUG** including what people call Traditional HERBS. And certainly VITAMINS and MINERALS and most other SUPPLEMENTS are just different versions of DRUGS.

REVOLUTIONARY HEALTH INSITE #129: **Many of the HEALTH FOOD STORES on the market today are essentially a FRONT for BIG PHARMA Drug Pushers**. In other words they are owned by the same people who SELL us PRESCRIPTION DRUGS (BAYER, MERCK, BASF, MONSANTO are all typically in bed with GNC, PHARMA VITE, SOLGARs of the world)!

REVOLUTIONARY HEALTH INSITE #130: **The STOMACH FLORA and DIGESTIVE FLORA rebuilds itself daily. And it is full of FAT (or MUCUOSA).** If you have IRRITABLE BOWEL SYNDROME, CELIAC, CROHNS or DIVERTICULITIS--all of these are signs of INFLAMMATION in the GUT--however, can be HEALED by the MUCOSA time to change and evolve. WHOLE FOODS, DISTILLED WATER and good OIL (virgin Coconut, Olive, Sesame Seed or Butter oils....depending your ETHNICITY) can help Heal this issue.

REVOLUTIONARY HEALTH INSITE #131: **If you are not FEELING well you may NOT be EATING the Proper FOODS for Your METABOLISM (and you may especially be low on PROTEIN or at least what we CALL proteins...for proteins is really just a made up word, however, we use it to communicate the point; likewise, the amount of CARBOHYDRDATES consumption may be too high).** Everyone METABOLIZES Food different. Some people are FAST METABOLIC TYPES and others are SLOW METABOLIC TYPES, which is known as FAST or SLOW OXIDATION (depends on HYPOTHALAMUS GLAND & WATER INTAKE determined by how often you Feel the need to Eat). Generally, most of us are on a Too High Carbs Diet which affects our entire BIOKHEMISTRY! Your best level of DENSE low, carbs will immediately improve well-being, energy and mood. When I say LOW—I simply mean LOW compared to someone else. Again everybody is different so your amount of CARBS may actually need to be HIGH in relation to the next person; and even LOWER compared to YET someone else!

REVOLUTIONARY HEALTH INSITE #132: **EATING is Less a Source of ENERGY to the HUMAN BODY than we realize.** And it is this WRONG misconception that informs our tendency to OVEREAT to the point of SICKNESS and DISEASE. Actually, Eating is a DRAIN on the ENERGY RESERVES of the body. This is why its kritical that we learn how to MAXIMIZE alternate energy pathways (FAT rather than SUGAR, for example, as well as utilizing the SUN, WATER, FASTING, DEEP BREATHING, EXERCISE and MEDITATION).

REVOLUTIONARY HEALTH INSITE #133: **What we Feed our MINDS** is just as Important as what we Feed our BODIES!

REVOLUTIONARY HEALTH INSITE #134: **A Body in GOOD HEALTH** is a GOD in HEAVEN. Great, nutritious eating actually induces a kind of EUPHORIA! Because you realize you are finally eating for YOUR particular CELLULAR TYPE. And not someone ELSE. There are only certain foods that can give you the Most BANG for the BITE. Find them and eat them and everyone of your CELLS will scream and holler in JOY. It is HEAVEN on EARTH!

REVOLUTIONARY HEALTH INSITE #135: **We must BREATHE DEEPLY, for it is our LUNGS which moves our LYMPH around. And it is the HEART that moves our BLOOD around. Both are important.** However, the LYMPH has NO Pump per se, rather it is Forced thru our bodies via the ACTION of the LUNGS. Thus, the DEEPER you BREATHE, the more LYMPH you generate throughout the body proper. And Lymph is where IMMUNITY resides. So please BREATHE DEEP!

REVOLUTIONARY HEALTH INSITE #136: **There is No such-a thang as a COMPLETE PROTEIN.** All PROTEINS are INCOMPLETE until they are RESTRUCTURED by the DIGESTIVE SYSTEM proper. So MEAT does not have MORE Complete Proteins than VEGS/FRUITS. Each ORGANIC food source has a PART of the Protein Puzzle that combines thru RITE eating. And this is how we get all the PROTEINS we need! Meat may have more ESSENTIAL AMINO ACIDS (so-called) which are PROTEINS; however, it still is not COMPLETE—as it takes ALL 22 Proteins to be truly complete and NO one TRUE food has that (protein shakes do not count—and even if they did the amount of SUGAR renders many of the available proteins useless)!

REVOLUTIONARY HEALTH INSITE #137: **One of your BEST protections against H1N1 is AVOIDING all CHICKENS, DUCKS and PORK Meats.** All of these animals have FILTHY habits and carry a GENETIC VARIANT of the H1N1 Strain. Additionally, their Preparation/Slaughter is UNSANITARY as well. Its NOT a FLU EPIDEMIC that we need to be careful of—it is a TAINTED MEAT PANDEMIC! It is the MEAT that has been compromised and the government is simply afraid to tell us the TRUTH about it!

REVOLUTIONARY HEALTH INSITE #138: **The DOCTRINE of SIGNATURES applies to MEAT as well as HERBS or FRUITS. The THEORY being that FRUITS/VEGETABLES are Shaped like the parts of the Body they can Heal. Same with MEAT!** For example, one should eat KIDNEYS for Kidney issues; LIVER for liver issues, PANCREAS for Pancreas issues; HEART for Heart issues; TESTICLES/PENIS/OVARIES for REPRODUCTIVE issues.

REVOLUTIONARY HEALTH INSITE #139: **CALCIUM is a JOKE—and a HUSTLE by the VITAMIN INDUSTRY (once again)! We have been OVERSOLD on taking CALCIUM as a Supplement. And in this form, mostly, LEECHES the Calcium OUT of our BONES rather than DEPOSITING it into them.** This is due to this Synthetic form of the Mineral being mostly useless ROCK! It cant be ABSORBED and therefore disturbs your BONE MATRIX (COLLAGEN, and so on). A better CURE for OSTEOPOROSIS is simple WEIGHT-BEARING activities like WEIGHT LIFTING (not too heavy tho), WALKING, BOUNDING (on small trampoline, for example), PLYOMETRICS and easy EXERCISES like PUSHUPS, PULLUPS, SITUPS (modified to fit your condition). Even better when these things are done outdoors in the SUN/HEAT.

In terms of a SUPPLEMENT that actually WORKS—you should go with one of the Powerful CLAYS such as BENTONITE, MONTORMORILLONITE or FULLERS EARTH (these are all DIFFERENT names for the same thing). CLAY is potent and has been used for thousands of years for all kinds of MEDICINAL reasons: BUILDING BONES, PREGNANCY <to supply CALCIUM>, CHELATION, RASHES, BOILS <a kind of MRSA>. Do NOT use MUCH for consumption purposes. Just a pinch will do you well. CLAY is EFFECTIVE and HEALING enough to be included in the UNITED STATES PHARMACOPEIA (USP) which is STANDARDS-SETTING watchdog for all PRESCRIPTION DRUGS, OVER THE COUNTER MEDICINES and SUPPLEMENTS (vitamins, minerals, herbs).

REVOLUTIONARY HEALTH INSITE #140: **BIOCHEMICALLY (what is going on inside the body), there is NO difference between ALCOHOL, HEROINE, COCAINE and----SUGAR!** All of them affect OPIOD RECEPTORS, levels of DOPAMINE and SEROTONIN (Brain Chemicals that control your EMOTIONS for HUMAN or ANIMALISTIC Behavior).

REVOLUTIONARY HEALTH INSITE #141: **URIC ACID is one of the most Powerful, Protective ANTIOXIDANT Nutrients for the Human Body--it just happens to be Abundant in MEAT!** However, this is a good thing, because its MORE ABSORBABLE from a MEAT SOURCE. As always EAT Ya MEAT like you eat your VEGETABLES: clean and organic as possible (example: Grassfed, Kosher, Organic, Halal). And there are other Antioxidants in Meat such as CARNOSINE. Both are implicated in long-lived people/species. Additionally, dont forget that in addition to DARK GREENS and VITAMIN C FRUITS--FATTY MEAT is also an IMMUNE BOOSTER! The KEY? Do Not GORGE yourself on Meat. A few ounces per 10-12 days. We must understand that when the SEASON changes it SHIFTS our body to more reliance on Antioxidant Protective SATURATED FATS, URIC ACID & CARNOSINE which are better ASSIMILATED from MEAT (or MEAT-BY PRODUCTS, ie., EGGS, BUTTER). *(See Insite #192).*

REVOLUTIONARY HEALTH INSITE #142: **Too many People are making a LIVING OFF THE CULTURE rather than CREATING SUSTAINABLE Culture.** Many are conducting themselves like VULTURESE on a CARCASS, PICKING it apart to line their POCKETS (and STOMACHS) with leftover DEAD Ideas and DISEASED THINKING and calling this PROGRESS. PROSPERITY (of the LAW of ATTRACTION) is mostly about ATTRACTING YOU to a SEMINAR SO YOU CAN pay them a LOT OF MONEY)!

REVOLUTIONARY HEALTH INSITE #143: **The FRANKENMEDS long ago figured out that the BRAIN could be Completely RE-WIRED (BRAINWASHED) simply by MANIPULATING the FOOD SUPPLY.** So here we stand on the brink of EXTINCTION because our MOUTHS have gotten us into trouble again! 12 NERVES *(VAGUS, OLFACTORY, GLOSSOPHARYNGEAL, OPTIC, OCULOMOTOR, TROCHLEAR, TRIGEMINAL, ABDUCENS, FACIAL, VESTIBULOCHLEAR, SPINAL ACCESSORY and HYPOGLOSSAL)* coming straight out of the CRANIUM, all connected to the TONGUE in some way should be a sober REMINDER how easy it is to STEAL the MINDS of a People thru TASTE alone! (REPTILES, for example, maintain this ability as they SENSE and SMELL with their tongues….and some would say we are just EVOLVED Reptiles—a REPTILIAN RACE)! *(see Insite #84).*

REVOLUTIONARY HEALTH INSITE #144: **MARATHONERS need to switch to FAT LOADING (rather than CARBO LOADING) if they want to finish the RACE in RECORD Times!** Therefore, CARB-LOADING as many Marathon Runners do is in error. Rather one should FAT LOAD! CARBOHYDRATES provide energy for the FIRST part of the race. This much is true, however, for the COMPLETION of the race—a RUNNER must have FAT STORES—not SUGAR, ie., GLUCOSE STORES from CARBS that is the current strategy. SPRINTERS, on the other hand, should be the ones who actually concentrate on CARBO-LOADING! They are the ones who need that GLUCOSE STORED up in their MUSCLES (for explosive ENERGY)!! The SPORTS INDUSTRY is EATING/FEEDING their athletes RONG.

REVOLUTIONARY HEALTH INSITE #145: **SKINNY, NERVOUS, HIGH STRUNG, ECTOMORPH-types need a LOW CARBOHYDRATE, HIGH FAT, HIGH PROTEIN Eating Regimen.** This is due to a High Carb Diet resulting in eating too much SUGAR which simply irritates your NERVES/NERVOUS SYSTEM, forcing you to EXHAUST your SYMPATHETIC NERVOUS SYSTEM, leading to CHRONIC FATIGUE. It also AGES you too quickly. This will keep you Sickly. You will be running off of Sugar when you need to be running off of FAT (which is more CALMING to the Nerves for SLIM/ECTOMORPH types because it results more in the use of your PARASYMPATHETIC NERVOUS SYSTEM).

REVOLUTIONARY HEALTH INSITE #146: **The reason so many of us are SICK is because we live life via our SYMPATHETIC NERVOUS SYSTEM (which codes for STRESS and uses the HORMONE that AGES us—INSULIN/CORTISOL); rather than our PARASYMPATHETIC NERVOUS SYSTEM (which uses the HORMONE that keeps us from AGING—GLUCAGON/DHEA).** This is why its so important that we learn to RELAX, bringing our PARASYMPATHETIC NERVOUS SYSTEM into play more than the SNS. Eastern Meditation is based on this principle even tho it does not say anything about this connection.

REVOLUTIONARY HEALTH INSITE #147: **VACCINATIONS cause your BODYs IMMUNE SYSTEM to shut down. The Innate Intelligence of the body reasons this from the foreign chemical that comes in via the Vaccination Shot that there is an outside source handling your IMMUNITY needs and therefore the BODY itself does NOT need to manufacture protective HORMONES or PROBIOTICS (not ANTIBIOTICS which mean AGAINST LIFE).** Even WITHOUT Vaccination, your body will MAKE its own PROBIOTIC to fite disease within 2-4 days on the short side; and 5-10 days on the long side. The CENTER FOR DISEASE CONTROL (CDC) tells us that 99% of AMERICANS will NOT be harmed by most of the FLU VIRUSES that are in existence INCLUDING the so-called PANDEMIC of the H1N1 (H1N1 HOAX I call it)! REPEAT: NOT HARMED. Thus, there is NO NEED to get VACCINATED against a DISEASE/FLU that 99% of us will NEVER get anyway—and if we do, even WITHOUT the SHOT—we will RECOVER in as little as 48 hours and certainly within 7-10 days (about as long as it takes to get a letter from AMERIKA to EUROPE).

REVOLUTIONARY HEALTH INSITE #148: **We must include both UNDER EATING and NO EATING in our FEEDING CYCLE for optimum health. At least 2 days of Under Eating; and 2 days of No Eating out of a total of 12 days (every CYCLE should be divided into 12 rather than the standard 7 day week).** This gives the BODY ample REST and RECUPERATION from the RAVAGES of eating. DIGESTING food uses up a lot of the STORED energy in the Body. Eating too OFTEN/MUCH leaves the body with METABOLIC RESIDUE in the bloodstream (food particles, especially from hard-to-digest items such as TRANSFATS, SUGAR, DRUGS, GRAINS). These can cause SEPSIS when it changes the PH BALANCE of the BLOOD.

REVOLUTIONARY HEALTH INSITE #149: **If you have a CHOICE (and can afford it) when it comes to getting "new teeth" go with a DENTAL TITANIUM/ZIRCONIUM TOOTH IMPLANT.** Its expensive, yet worth it because it helps keep that JAWBONE (and Nerves of the face) alive moreso than getting DENTURES or BRIDGE WORK. Furthermore, A Tooth EXTRACTION is essentially SURGERY! The body then sends extra HEALING to that location. Thus, whenever a TOOTH is pulled the BALANCE of the body on that side of the body is upset.

REVOLUTIONARY HEALTH INSITE #150: **The WEED of today is TAINTED with so many PESTICIDES that it is turning MEN into WOMEN and WOMEN into MEN because the chemicals are HORMONE DISRUPTERS!!** Some of us have higher levels of THC in our BRAINS and when this ENDOGENOUS (cause its inside the body) chemical mixes with the THC in Weed—it stimulates an OVERPRODUCTION of the normal amount of THC at the CANNABINOID RECEPTORS in the Brain! This causes you to go overboard. This constantly repeated process winds up killing off Brain cells rather CREATING more New Cells (a process called NEUROGENESIS). This leads to developing DISEASE symptoms of ALZHEIMER (this aint just Weed forgetting—this is serious BRAIN CELLS being lost)! PARKINSONS, MULTIPLE SCLEROSIS and other diseases that destroy the NERVOUS SYSTEM start showing up as well. Factor in extreme PARANOIA, SCHIZOPHRENIA and INSANITY and you have the recipe for a true KILLER WEED! Thus, it should be noted that NO other ETHNICAL group has more THC at those CANNIBINOID RECEPTORS than People of COLOR! Therefore, this makes Weed particularly DANGEROUS for these cultures of people.

Likewise, this WEED of today has a ESTROGEN/TESTOSTERONE switch in them, meaning they flip ESTROGEN to TESTOSTERONE and TESTOSTERONE to ESTROGEN! This causes a SWAP out of your GENES via those HORMONAL PATHWAYS!! All of sudden as a MAN you get the urge to SUCK a PENIS and you wont know why! BLAME it on the WEED. You are a WOMAN who develops a rather OVERDEVELOPED interest in eating COOCHIE! BLAME YA WEED!

Simply put: nowadays WEED is more of a DESTROYER of the Brain than a BENEFIT! It is a DETRIMENT not a BENEFIT. We need to understand this: And as with the GENDER BENDERing with WEED—this is also happening with other HYPNOGOGIC/PSYCHOTIC drugs they are using with PATIENTS! Additionally, the PESTICIDES like PARAQUAT that have been and are used on WEED is extremely dangerous (after all WEED is just another CROP like any other)......All from these NEW KHEMICALS they are using to grow the crops SUPER FAST!

SIDENOTE: WEED stopped being good after the 1970s when the GOVERNMENT decided it was time to stop using the DRUG on Soldiers and MK ULTRA programs and start selling it to the public for PROFIT. Many old heads, in fact, think thatz what VIETNAM was about really: DRUGS. Both the MARIJUANA and HEROIN trades benefitted from the VIETNAM WAR. Indeed. Drugs are always involved in these wars: KOREAN WAR had OPIUM at its foundation. And the current war in IRAQ is about OPIUM, HASH, HEROIN and MARIJUAN (HEMP). Same difference. Nothing has changed yawl!

REVOLUTIONARY HEALTH INSITE #151: **The THYROID is the FURACE of the body and must be kept FIRED UP with its Fuel—IODINE!** No Iodine means NO FIRE. And No fire means COLD. As in COLDS, FLUS, SICKNESS—and basically, NO IMMUNITY! They THYROID contains the SPIRITUAL HEAT of the body and if it goes out—the BODY itself goes out! It works in cooperation with the *THYMUS* which must have ZINC to keep it LIT.

REVOLUTIONARY HEALTH INSITE #152: **HOMOSEXUALITY (GAY/LESBIANISM) is a BIRTH DEFECT like any other disease—and as such can be REVERSED and/or HEALED.** Thatz provided a person WANTS to be Healed. Some do not. And thatz their rite. The KEY like most other things are in your DIET and your THINKING (metaphysics aspect).

So yes, a CHILD can be BORN GAY due to overproduction of ESTROGEN (male) or TESTOSTERONE (female) during CONCEPTION. For example, DOKTORS have already shown that the SEX ORIENTATION of an animal can be CHANGED in the WOMB! (even up to the Third TRIMESTER)! Thus, this is/can be a BIRTH DEFECT as noted (or CONCEPTUS INTERRUPTUS, if you will). If the MAMA does not have proper FOODS while carrying her child—it can be affected in the womb. Especially, the rite and proper amounts of FATS (lecithin, for example), VITAMIN K, IRON and so on. Fats are critical as they help make the PROPER amount of HORMONES that the child needs to be the MALE or FEMALE they are SUPPOSED to be!! Likewise, SUGAR is a Huge DISRUPTER of the correct Distribution of said Hormones (or any DRUG for that matter). Many women have a residual effect of BIRTH HORMONES left over in their REPRODUCTIVE ORGANS and this too can ALTER your childs GENES!!(METHYLATION).

Knowing this means that the GENES of your child can be SWITCHED back to their Proper SETTING with the right FOODS and MENTAL COUNSELING (depending on what AGE the child is).

REVOLUTIONARY HEALTH INSITE #153: **The VEGAN/VEGETARIAN lifestyle is NOT for BLACK people or People of COLOR!** Yes, there are some EXCEPTIONS. And they are just that: EXCEPTIONS! The DIGESTIVE TRACK of COLORED people is not meant to eat the DIET of HERBIVORES, exclusively: All PLANT FOODS, ALL THE TIME! The HYDROCHLORIC ACID in our stomachs is able to change to meet the types of foods we MUST eat to survive: PLANTS, SEEDS, NUTS, DAIRY or MEAT! This is nothing new: this is something ANCIENT! AYURVEDIC (FOOD as) MEDICINE! We are OMINVOROUS Beings. Not just a MONO DIET eating SPECIES. If we were only meant to eat PLANTS only—we would have ADAPTED to have EYES on the sides of our HEADS ala ELEPHANTS, ZEBRAS, GIRAFFES, FISH and so on (some exceptions include the SHARK who are MEAT-eaters, yet as a result of that type of eating—they are pure KILLERS). Additionally, these HERBIVOROUS ANIMALS are PREY (read: FOOD) for other PREDATORY animals. Humans are not. If we were meant to eat MEAT only we would have CANINE TEETH. We do not. *(see Insite #0).*

REVOLUTIONARY HEALTH INSITE #154: **Severe CRAVINGS are how Your body signals you to find an appropriate FOOD SOURCE for the Deficient NUTRIENT.** Preferably, LIVE, WHOLE FOODS, NUTRIENT-DENSE ones to RE-SUPPLY the Mineral. Constant Cravings mean you are NOT addressing the NUTRIENT NEED correctly. For example: you may be eating too many REFINED/PROCESSED foods and suffering from MALNUTRITION as a result. This is what gives many people a Dis-ease called PICA (a craving for weird things such as PASTE, DIRT, TOBACCO, LEAD and so on). Your body is looking for the MINERALS and/or the ELEMENTAL Metals contained within these inorganic items—that you NEED to OBTAIN from real, LIVE, WHOLE, NUTRIENT-DENSE foods. However, most of us will simply eat Refined Foods or take SYNTHETIC vitamins that STILL do not SUPPLY the body with the Nutrient. Mainly because these items or fake foods do not break down into a form that can get inside the BLOOD CELL and be used!

REVOLUTIONARY HEALTH INSITE #155: **Most of our BONE LOSS leading to OSTEOPOROSIS comes from eating REFINED CARBOHYDRATES/PROCESSED FOODS and SUGAR.** Both of these FAKE FOODS leech VITAMIN D, density from the Bones and the TEETH.

REVOLUTIONARY HEALTH INSITE #156: **The LONGEST-LIVED People in the world ALL eat MEAT!** In fact, MEAT EATERS live just as long as VEGANS or VEGETARIANS. The key is to eat meat in MODERATION. No more than 10-20% of your EATIQUETTE (diet). Thus, 2-4 days out of 12 would be sufficient to consume Meat and obtain its benefits WITHOUT "taxing" your body. The idea that being just a VEGAN will help you live longer than a Moderate Meat eater is a LIE. Plenty of Vegans/Vegetarians DIE of CANCER and other DISEASES (mostly because many of them are MALNOURISHED....and a BODY without proper Nutrients will DECAY and PASS AWAY)!!

REPEATING: As far as it is known in the modern era, the LONGEST LIVED people in the world ALL--I repeat ALL----EAT MEAT! *Not much Meat* (which is what I recommend, personally, as less than 10-20% of your DIETS, same as these LONG LIVED folks----*but they DO EAT it*....and have been eating it for MILLENNIA). And thatz what we are MISSING about this whole thing. A little MEAT every once in a while is not going to RUIN your HEALTH. In fact, it will enhance it due to the URIC ACID content of the Meat. Just eat your Meat CLEAN. Its worth going through the trouble of finding good, organic, cleaner meats for the HEALTH benefits. WE miss the POINT that most of our SOCIETIES thrived from mixing up their DIETS consisting of "both" MEAT and VEGETABLES. As well as FRUITS, SEEDS, NUTS, WATER and FAT. We need to be careful of these extreme MONO DIETS that the HEALTH INDUSTRY keeps SELLING people on. Especially, my BLACK bretheren and sistren need to be careful of VEGAN diets (in general, they are not for the BLACK Man and Woman....why? because we have HIGHER nutritional requirements due to CARBON, ie, Melanin....we need more GLUCOSE, SODIUM, hell even SUN than most other

ETHNIC types....and for most of us PLANTS and FRUITS while DEFINITELY beneficial need to be SUPPLEMENTED with MEAT, at the least, FISH). Thus, the NATURAL DIET of HUMANS is Not just PLANTS, ie., VEGETABLES or FRUIT. It also includes SEEDS, NUTS and MEAT. And yes, WATER. Even AIR and SUN must be INHALED as a Normal part of what we consume. We are not HERBIVORES. We are OMNIVORES. We are not just CARNIVORES. We are OMNIVORES. *In fact, If you want to be TECHNICAL about it--based on PHYSIOLOGY, the "natural" diet of Humans would be SUNLITE (thatz why you have a SOLAR plexus; and a digestive COLON meaning SUN!!). However, letz not be TECHNICAL shall we? Letz just be PRACTICAL based on the world we are living in today. With all the STRESSES, HATERS of modern living. For that you need--should i say it? a little MEAT! Come on now. Just a little bite off the corner of an organic piece of BEEF aint gonna KILL ya! About er' 10-12 days will HEAL you.*

REVOLUTIONARY HEALTH INSITE #157: **How is that so many so-called CONSERVATIVES are TOLERANT of the BANK BAILOUT and the CAR INDUSTRY BAILOUT? Yet, are upset that President BARACK OBAMA is proposing a HEALTHCARE SYSTEM that would BAIL OUT our own AMERIKAN CITIZENRY? So its OK to ensure the HEALTH of the BANKS and CARS--but NOT the PEOPLE?!** Ironically, the BANK/CAR Bailouts were never intended to Work. However, the PEOPLE ARE (expected to WORK). They caint work if they are bankrupted from lack of HEALTHCARE.

CONSERVATIVES like to say OBAMAs plan will just result in more DEBT for its hardworking CITIZENS. NOT TRUE when you actually dig deep into it: under OBAMAS longterm plan, NO DEBT would be passed onto the CITIZENS. Thatz a MYTH. In fact, DEBT would be LIFTED from the Citizens and placed where it belongs: in the HANDS of the GOVERNMENT! The CRITICS call this SOCIALIZED MEDICINE as tho it's a 4-letter word. Yet, in countries where it exists—the PEOPLE are HEALTHIER and LONGER-LIVED overall! (JAPAN and SWITZERLAND, for example). Meanwhile, under the current HEALTHCARE SYSTEM—here in the UNITED STATES, the RICHEST country in the world—we rank at the BOTTOM of industrialized countries in terms of WELLNESS for our people!

REVOLUTIONARY HEALTH INSITE #158: **Overcome INFERTILITY to Create a SUPER BABY in this manner: the number one NUTRIENT for parents who want a FANTASTIK FETUS should be ZINC for the MAN; and IRON for the WOMAN. This ZINC should come from a FOOD such as SUNFLOWER SEEDS; and the IRON should come from a MAMMAL such as COW BEEF (even if you are a VEGAN).** Its KRITICAL to get ELEMENTAL MINERALS from your Food Sources otherwise, there can NOT be proper Assimilation of Nutrients into the CELLS. And without this—NO potential SUPER CHILD can come forth! There are other kritical nutrients too including IODINE, FAT, VITAMIN A, VITAMIN B, VITAMIN C, VITAMIN E, VITAMIN D, VITAMIN K (for the Woman); and SELENIUM, MAGNESIUM, ZINC, CHLOROPHYLL (for the Man). Of course, GENDER, BLOODTYPE, LOCATION & ETHNICITY come into play (so me for a consultation for more insite into that).

Additionally, NITE TIME is the Best Time to EAT (in general) and day time is the best time for SEX/REPRODUCTION. However, if you want to INCREASE your chances of a GIRL child make love in the DAYLITE; and if you want to INCREASE your chances of a BOY child make love at NITE TIME! Your CIRCADIAN RHYTHM (see that entry) may be different, of course. If so, MAKE LOVE according to your CR.

However, the PARASYMPATHETIC NERVOUS SYSTEM comes online more at night making it more useful for eating and DIGESTING (food) and RESTING *(see Insite #22).*

Whereas when it comes to making BABIES: to increase your chances of having a GIRL have SEX in the DAYTIME. However, if you want to increase your chances of having a BOY—get busy with it in the NITE TIME (preferably, on a FULL MOON). This is because the IONS of the NITE AIR are MASCULINE/YANG in nature. While those of the PHOTONS of the Day Air (SUN) are FEMININE/YIN in nature. In fact, the SUN *is* FEMININE (NOT masculine as we have been sold), thus is why MORE Girls are born in certain parts of the world (ie., the CARRIBEAN, the ISLANDS, around the EQUATOR where the SUN is more prevalent....and MORE Girls are also born during the SUMMER months when more DAYLITE; and more Boys are born during the WINTER when more NITELITE).

SIDENOTE: A good Natural baby FOOD for a CHILD is SUNFLOWER SEED MILK/CEREAL is GREAT. Boil RAW Sunflower Seeds FEW minutes. Pour off HOT WATER. BLEND using DISTILLED WATER as needed to THICKEN/THIN. BABY can eats this once a month. DENSE amounts of FAT, PROTEIN, CALCIUM, VITAMIN D, IRON and HYDROGEN contained within! The CHILD only needs to eat a little to benefit.

REVOLUTIONARY HEALTH INSITE #159: **CHRONIC FATIGUE is a Dis-ease of Using the Rong NERVOUS SYSTEM. This is because the Body runs off 2 Nervous Systems: SYMPATHETIC and PARASYMPATHETIC.** The use of the SYMPATHETIC NERVOUS SYSTEM is much HARDER on the body than the PARASYMPATHETIC NERVOUS SYSTEM. And if you are primarily using SYMPATHETIC, then, your body is in a CONSTAT state of TURMOIL which leads to ILLNESS and lack of IMMUNITY. Thus, at the BROAD level, most any DIS-EASE you are dealing with is ROOTED in your SYMPATHETIC Nervous being Exhausted. Conversely, your return to HEALTH is rooted in AWAKENING your PARASYMPATHETIC Nervous System to assist in HEALING you.

REVOLUTIONARY HEALTH INSITE #160: **To paraphrase the Hon. ELIJAH MUHAMMAD--Do NOT ever eat REFINED CARBOHYDRATES** even if you have to STARVE TO DEATH!

REVOLUTIONARY HEALTH INSITE #161: **The BODY is REGENERATED by the NITE IONS in the MOONLITE!** Due to the amount of MELANIN, IRON and COPPER stored in your CELLS (going forward towards 2012 these ELEMENTS must be increased in our EATING REGIMENS). This is why its just as important to MOON BATHE as it is to SUN BATHE.

REVOLUTIONARY HEALTH INSITE #162: **Your BLOODCELLS store Information based on the VIBRATION of your HEARTBEAT. They read this Beat much like the ANCIENTS read the sounds of the DRUMS thru a RIVER (BLOOD is the RIVER OF LIFE indeed)! This is why its extremely important that STRESS is avoided by the production of excess CORTISOL and INSULIN**—because your Heart sends such Khemical DISTRESS signals to your BloodCells who then carry this MESSAGE to all the ORGANS of the Body proper. Such a constant signal will EXHAUST your Organs, especially, your HEART and PANCREAS, leading to HEART ATTACK (STOPPAGE) and DIABETES (Sugar Crash).

REVOLUTIONARY HEALTH INSITE #163: **As KRAZY as it may seem--SOME of us NEED a few ACHES and PAINS to keep us MOTIVATED towards HEALTH!** Without such SIGNALS many of would not even *MONITOR* our HEALTH!

REVOLUTIONARY HEALTH INSITE #164: **As a RULE, avoid DIETARY SUPPLEMENTS because they can actually MUTATE our GENES: switching OFF those that HELP us; and switching ON those that HARM us (this is called METHYLATION)!** Therefore, we need to be extremely careful in taking these VITAMINS/MINERALS without proper guidance. We must never forget that these Nutrients are just a different class of DRUGS (without a PRESCRIPTION)! Furthermore, ALWAYS buy the most EXPENSEIVE, BEST QUALITY Supplement you can afford from one of those INDIVIDUAL, Renegade-type DOCTORS *(like Dr. SEBI, Dr. PAUL GOSS, Dr. BOB MARSHALL, Dr. RAYMOND FRANCIS, Dr. RUSSELL BLAYLOCK & Dr. JOSEPH MERCOLA).* The day of the VITAMIN STORE is gone! To ensure quality control, go with a LONE doctor. Especially good are those who were once a part of the establishment and have decided to turn their backs on the medical industry now! *(see Insite#65).*

REVOLUTIONARY HEALTH INSITE #165: **The Human Body should never be CUT OPEN because this lets too much OXYGEN out of the body. Rather SURGERY should always be done through the NATURAL OPENINGS (ORIFICES) of the body proper** (the NOSE, RECTUM, EYES, ARMPITS, NAVEL, PENIS<Men>, VAGINA<women>, MOUTH and EARS). Additionally, you DISTURB the Nerves and the Energy levels of the body at the Site of the CUT. Better ALTERNATIVES are ACCUNPUNCTURE, ACCUPRESSURE, MASSAGE, MOVMENT are all supposed to be used to RESTORE Energy to the body. Some say the body would have a ZIPPER on it if it was meant to be OPENED. Of course, NO ZIPPER--however, if one just has to INVADE the body it does has at least 10 NATURAL OPENINGS that can be used rather than CUTTING it up!! 2 EYES, 2 EARS, 2 NOSTRILS, 1 MOUTH, 1 NAVEL, 1 RECTUM, 1 PENIS=10 OPENINGS. All of these NATURAL ORIFICES can be used to ENTER the Body for any sort of operation. If they can not be used then this means that the DISEASE is not THAT serious—and can HEAL on its own!!

This is why the work of DOCTORS in countries like INDIA who are practicing NATURAL ORIFICE Non-Cut Surgery are leading the way to NON-INVASIVE SURGERY. Amerikan FRANKENMEDS do not trust it and thus CRITICIZE it, calling it PRIMITIVE and BACKWARDS. Which means they can not make enuff MONEY off of it! Every part of the INTERNAL workings of the body can be reached thru these Naturally provided openings put there by NATURE/CREATOR. Amerika is behind even so-called 3rd world countries in Medical Advances/Thinking).

REVOLUTIONARY HEALTH INSITE #166: **PROTEIN can not be Absorbed properly from every form of Food by the DIGESTIVE TRACK. Altho it is in everything including even a ROCK.** Yet, Humans have a hard time absorbing in the most efficient way from, say, VEGETABLES or FRUITS only. To get more of the Protein Nutrient, other foods like MEAT, SEEDS, NUTS, EGGS, CHEESE have to be included in your EATING. This allows the BODY to Complete more of the PROTEIN PUZZLE.

REVOLUTIONARY HEALTH INSITE #167: **Take VITAMIN B and C together.** They move in the BLOOD and the LYMPH SYSTEM (Lymphatic Fluid). Very important to the LYMPHATIC SYSTEM, especially in terms of AUTO-IMMUNE diseases. Addressing NERVES, HAIR, SKIN, EYES, LIVER and PANCREAS. Helps with INSULIN.

REVOLUTIONARY HEALTH INSITE #168: **You Must EAT (and DRINK) NATURAL FOODS that RESONATE with You; those Foods that you have a CRAVING for and that are WHOLE, LIVE and PROTEIN/NUTRIENT-DENSE.** Even though these particular foods are Not GOOD for anyone else. They are the PERFECT ones for YOU! Those are the foods that will SUSTAIN and give you the Longest LIFESPAN.

REVOLUTIONARY HEALTH INSITE #169: **Best NATURAL DEFENSE to COLDS, FLUS is to FAST.** Thereby allowing your BODYs natural defenses to come to your RESCUE and and FITE for you.

REVOLUTIONARY HEALTH INSITE #170: **FREE RADICALS cause OXIDATION (RUST) because IRON is the NUCLEUS of your CELLS!** And what does OXYGEN do to IRON? Rite! It causes RUST! However, you can provide your CELLS with a layer of LIPID (fat) by consuming good, organic OILS (Thinner <Olive Oil> ones in the Summer; Thicker <Coconut Oil> ones in the Winter as a general rule).

REVOLUTIONARY HEALTH INSITE #171: **KANCER can be prevented in most places of the Body by keeping CERTAIN NUTRIENTS flowing thru the BODY: For example, the IODINE stores of the THYROID must be up to par (thus TOMATOES, CELERY; and supplementation where needed with LUGOLS or IODORALS).** And you need VITAMIN C and LITHIUM (from LEMONS) which are 2 of the most critical nutrients in the history of HUMANKIND!! And especially in the general PREVENTION of CANCER. Also need SILICON/SILICA (CUCUMBERS). Need IRON so the LIVER can be strong. LACTOFERRIN is crucial (CHEESE, FERMENTED DAIRY PRODUCTS). The KIDNEYS/BLOODSTREAM need small amounts of URIC ACID (eating LAMB/GOAT KIDNEYS or BEEF will supply this or as a supplement where necessary—Baby ASPIRIN or IODIZED SEA SALT); ADRENAL GLANDS need ELECTRICITY (UVB RAYS/SUN).

REVOLUTIONARY HEALTH INSITE #172: **MEAT also has its DOCTRINE of SIGNATRES which states that a FOOD looks like the part of the body it will HEAL.** Usually we think of this with HERBS or PLANTS or VEGETABLES. However, the same can be said of MEAT. Thus, KIDNEYS for KIDNEYS; LIVER for LIVER, OVARIES/TESTICLES for Ovaries or Testicles; HEART for the HEART. NEVER, EVER EAT THE BRAIN of any ANIMAL, however!

REVOLUTIONARY HEALTH INSITE #173: OLEIC OIL (**Peanuts, Sesame Seed Oil) can be used to CURE all kinds of KANCER** (especially, of the ORGANS....THYROID or LIVER cancer, for example) because it STIMULATES the production of TUMOR NECROSIS FACTOR. This Factor is the BODYs own chemical that TURNS OFF the ONCOGENIC (cancerous) Gene. OLEIC OIL produces a khemical smell inside the body proper that signals CELL DEATH of dying tissue and stimulates other healthy cells to get rid of the DEAD CELLS before they DECAY, causing a poisonous gas to be released in the cavities of the body. This is how INSECTS also know to remove their own dead from the HIVE (Bees) or NEST (Ants). This is NECROSIS FACTOR at work. The P53 GENE works by this process, as it is a REGULATORY Gene that signals repair of other DAMAGED genes in the body—especially, the LIVER.

REVOLUTIONARY HEALTH INSITE #174: **Turn BAD PASTEURIZED MILK into GOOD MILK by adding APPLE CIDER VINEGAR to it.** This LIBERATES the Nutrients which are locked into the PASTEURIZED FAT, allowing them to be more readily absorbed by your CELLS. Also this creates beneficial bacterial GUT FLORA.

REVOLUTIONARY HEALTH INSITE #175: **A most KRITICAL Nutrient for BLACK people is TRYPTOPHAN and TYROSINE** due their ability to help make SEROTONIN, MELATONIN and PIGMENTATION *(indicated in cases of VITILIGO, for example)* a Hormone that helps you make BABIES and SLEEP. These Hormones help you to: DONT WORRY, BE HAPPY. The importance of these NUTRIENTS finds their strength especially in the WINTER when SEROTONIN levels can drop drastically; also in those dealing with ADDICTION issues from regular STREET DRUGS, SUGAR and/or PRESCRIPTION MEDS. Likewise, any TRAUMATIC EMOTIONAL situations can use up your Stores of TRYPTOPHAN and TYROSINE. Find it in BEEF, BISON, TURKEY, FISH, CHICKPEAS, CHEESE, GOAT MILK, YOGURT, CHOCOLATE, DURIANS, DATES, EGGS, PEANUTS, SUNFLOWER SEEDS and PUMPKIN SEEDS just to name some. Indeed, MELATONIN mite just be the most critical of all our BRAIN hormones as it is a SUPER POTENT ANTIOXIDANT as well. And may be the MAIN reason BLACK people live so long. It reduces the RAVAGES of FREE RADICAL brought on by STRESS! The BLACK BODY is under an INVISIBLE, yet very REAL type of POST TRAUMATIC SLAVE DISTRESS.

REVOLUTIONARY HEALTH INSITE #176: **The most critical Nutrient for WHITE PEOPLE is PHOSPHOROUS** which is found predominately in the BONE MATRIX where it helps to shore up that CALCIUM via HYDROXYAPATITE synthesis. Very important since our white bretheren have WEAKER bones that tend to HOLLOW OUT faster! This is also key for HEAD FRACTURES and CELL SIGNALING in the brain of White people leading to NEUROGENESIS (new brain cell growth...a good preventative to ALZHEIMERS). Find PHOSPHOROUS in SARDINES, FISH (like COD, MACKAREL, ORANGE ROUGHY), RAW MILK, CLAY, BAKING SODA (non-aluminum). You do not want PHOSPHATES/PHOSPHOROUS derived from SODAS, JUICES and HIGH FRUCTOSE CORN SYRUP products.

REVOLUTIONARY HEALTH INSITE #177: **Eat COLOSTRUM whenever you can! As a form of PROBIOTIC it is better than YOGURT alone because it contains more of the BIRTH/EMBRYONIC ENZYMES (ala BIFIDOBACTERIUM INFANTIS and BIFIDOBACTERIUM LONGUM which are bacteria that are present at your birth) at influencing NATAL and CHILDHOOD IMMUNITY longterm. Likewise, with BETA GLUCANS (example, Mushrooms and Brewers Yeast): also a powerful STIMULUS of EMBRYONIC STEM CELLS!** And this goes towards helping the DIGESTIVE TRACK generate more of the live, MICROORGANISMS that it needs to keep you Healthy. Very important considering 80% (inclusive of 4-pounds of BENEFICAL BACTERIA) of the IMMUNITY for the body is located in the DIGESTIVE TRACK! In terms of PROBIOTIC activity, the 2 most crucial BACTERIA to have in your DIGESTIVE SYSTEM are BIFIDOBACTERIUM INFANTIS and BIFIDOBACTERIUM LONGUM. So always look for PROBIOTICS that contain them.

REVOLUTIONARY HEALTH INSITE #178: **The level of CRIMINAL BEHAVIOR and INSANITY is because the BODY is not getting the NUTRIENTS it needs, especially, the B-VITAMINS such as B-6 (Pyridoxal Phosphate) and B-1 (Thiamine).** The B-Family of Vitamins influence the NERVOUS SYSTEM greatly, especially, the SYMPATHETIC NERVOUS SYTEM which helps to reign in BEHAVIOR. When the SNS takes charge too much of the body—DIS-EASES have an easier time manifesting due to the IMMUNE SYSTEM being broken down. B-VITAMINS help the IMMUNE SYSTEM function at its optimum. Thus, without B-Vitamins in the NERVOUS SYSTEM proper—Emotions and Behavior gets out of control, leading to all kinds of STRESS, OUTBURSTS and WEIRD behavior. Even MONSTROUS behavior (think GANGS/ORGANIZATIONS that rule the world like RELIGION, POLITICAL GROUPS rite on down to your local MAFIA; as well as personages such as the JEFFREY DAHMERS and JOHN WAYNE GACYs of society).

REVOLUTIONARY HEALTH INSITE #179: **NUTRIGENOMICS: The FACT that different ETHNIC GROUPS all get certain DISEASES that seem to be more ABUNDANT only amongst that certain Group is PROOF that we ALL have to EAT an INDIVIDUAL, PERSONALIZED Diet!** No 2 ETHNICITIES can eat the same. Hell, NO 2 People either! This is called NUTRIGENOMICS (NUTRINETICS): Eating for "YOUR" GENOME, down to ya GENE/BLOODCELL itself! And the HEALING TREATMENT must address this too. This goes toward the idea POLYMORPHISMS which are the VARIANTS we all have at the GENETIC level that contributes to our Individuality. These POLYMORPHISMS code for various micro differences in how we must EAT; who we are ETHNICALLY, who we are GENDERwise; and even where we must LIVE Geographically in order to Maintain WHOLENESS and WELLNESS!

REVOLUTIONARY HEALTH INSITE #180: **The KEY to making a SUPERBABY is for the WOMAN to consume IRON, B-COMPLEX, WATER and OIL; and the most important NUTRIENTS for the man to consume are ZINC, SELENIUM, IODINE and CHLROPHYLL.** These Nutrients are structured according to the WEIGHT of the CHROMOSOMES intent, ie., that the man supplies the CHILD with most of the IMMUNITY; while the woman supplies the child with most of its INTELLIGENCE.

REVOLUTIONARY HEALTH INSITE #181: **If you NEVER Bought another SUPPLEMENT the rest of your LIFE--there are still enough FOODS in your local FARMERS MARKET** to HEAL any DISEASE you may have to deal with. Just make sure to buy them ORGANIC when and where you can. If you can not, simply take them home and watch them. And in some cases let them SOAK overnite.

REVOLUTIONARY HEALTH INSITE #182: **ASPARTAME (is a chemical Poison) however, with its high PHENYLALANINE, FORMIC ACID content—it can be used to cure KANCER (Kidney, Liver, or Prostate, for example).** It helps produce a form of TUMOR NECROSIS FACTOR ALPHA which is a natural CYTOKINE of the body that SUPPRESSES CANCANCEROUS TUMORS (ala P53)! *Found in SODAS (however, drinking them is NOT the answer)!!* Obviously, it has to be part of a FORMULA. FORMIC ACID is a PHEROMONE/SALIVA used by ANTS to signal one another and to MARK territory—as well as to CLEANSE their environment by acting as a BACTERIAL ANTISEPTIC. We find a similar INGREDIENT with BEES and their PROPOLIS (ROYAL JELLY).

REVOLUTIONARY HEALTH INSITE #183: **The body cannot process PLASTIC or CARDBOARD. Yet, this is EXACTLY what we EAT** when we consume HYDROGENATED OIL, TRANSFATS or REFINED CARBOHYDRATES (Grains/Flour).

REVOLUTIONARY HEALTH INSITE #184: **FRUITS carry FRUIT SALTS; and VEGETABLES carry VEGETABLE SALTS. Both are needed for different reasons.** The SALTS of Fruit nourish more the ORGANS of the body; while the SALTS of Vegetables nourish more the BONES/JOINTS/TENDONS/LIGAMENTS of the body. Of course, there is overlap and Salts of each nourish ALL parts of the HUMAN PLANT as well. Thus, for, say, a LIVER dysfunction (Fatty Liver, Hepatitis) you want FRUIT SALTS; for a MUSCLE/JOINT/BONE dysfunction (Tendonitis, Arthritis) you want VEGETABLE SALTS.

REVOLUTIONARY HEALTH INSITE #185: **The BLADDER and KIDNEYS are the PETRI DISHES in the body.** Thus, its important to Keep them CLEAN so that an INFECTION does not build up in the Dish. For that you need a HIGH Vitamin C content in your FOODS. Also WATER, SEA SALT and IODINE. In fact, its good to drink WARM WATER and Sea Salt together (1/2 teaspoon to 16-20 ounces of water once a week as a maintenance drink).

REVOLUTIONARY HEALTH INSITE #186: **If you can Not SLEEP because your MIND is RACING at nite like you can not turn off your thoughts; you need more SEROTONIN/MELATONIN so consume TRYPTOPHAN** which can be made by eating such Foods as CHEESE, TURKEY, LECITHIN, EGGS & CHEESE together; or even GRAPES & CHEESE together. These foods help the body to Make TYRPTOPHAN which is a PRECURSOR to Serotonin and Melatonin. Essential to everyone; however, this nutrient is truly CRITICAL to all BLACK persons on the PLANET because it buffers STRESS and works hand in hand with *TYROSINE* (another critical nutrient) that helps Synthesize MELANIN—and even PIGMENTATION (VITILIGO, for example, can be helped with TYROSINE).

REVOLUTIONARY HEALTH INSITE #187: **ALZHEIMERS DISEASE is caused more by LACK of the key Nutrient: CHOLESTEROL than AMYLOID BETA PLACK or TANGLES (although that is the current theory).** You can get rid of the Plack/Tangles and STILL have the ALZHEIMERS. You will find that many with AD do not have ENOUGH Cholesterol or a dysfunction of the CHOLESTEROL via the LIVER.—thus THIS IS THE REAL PROBLEM: NO CHOLESTEROL!! For the LIVER and the BRAIN are connected. And if not enuff Cholesterol is being made thru the Synergy of the Liver—this can and will affect the BRAIN for worse, helping to BUILD UP the AMYLOID BETA PLACK which shows up as a PROTECTIVE MECHANISM much like CHOLESTEROL does itself in the VASCULAR SYSTEM proper. Change your Eating to include more CHOLESTEROL—and the problem of such DISEASES like AD can be prevented and HELPED (even HEALED)! DAIRY products: BUTTER, RAW GOAT/COW MILKS, EGGS, VIRGIN COCONUT OIL.

Additionally, PROBLEMS with the DIGESTIVE TRACK lead to many of the Most NEURODEGENERATIVE DISEASES like MULTIPLE SCLEROSIS, PARKINSONS, LOU GHERIGS and ALZHEIMERS because many MICRONUTRIENTS are not being ABSORBED (ie., COPPER, MOLYBDENUM, VANADIUM, BORON; and Hormones such as CHOLESTEROL (in the case of ALZHEIMERS). The ROOT STRUCTURE of the Digestive Track (which connects to the BRAIN STEM via the SPINAL CORD) becomes disconnected slightly causing a disruption in the NERVOUS PULSES going between the BRAIN and the DIGESTIVE TRACK in an Alternating Current. And this breakdown in communication can cause MEMORY LOSS, SHAKING, TREMORS and other Nervous Disorders. A Diet of consisting high SUGAR and REFINED CARBOHYDRATES (foods in which there are

NO/LITTLE nutrients) creates this MALNUTRITION; couple this with AGING and lack of HYDROCHLORIC ACID in the stomach and you have further uptake blockage of Nutrients—and ensuing DEFICIENCY.

MICRONUTRIENTS such as COPPER (which CONDUCTS the Nervous System proper) can be Deleted over time with a Diet devoid of live, whole Nutrients. Most of these smaller, micro nutrients are small and generally last a long time. However, once they are LOW in the TISSUES (body proper) they can cause HEALTH issues such as PARKINSONS and ALZHEIMERS which are NERVOUS SYSTEM-oriented. The REMEDY for this is to REPLACE these Nutrients over a long period of time along, including adequate OILS (to rebuild the MYELIN SHEATHS).

REVOLUTIONARY HEALTH INSITE #188: **The FRUITS that contribute MOST to the IMMUNITY of the Body are those that have SOUR and/or a SOUR "and" a SWEET taste.** For example: POMEGRANATES, LEMONS, LIMES, KIWI, APPLES, GREEN APPLES, BERRIES, STRAWBERRIES, ORANGES, NECTARINES, PLUMS, APRICOTS, PEACHES, PEARS, MANGOS. The SOURness of these fruits are what make for BACTERIA-genesis in the GUT, helping them to act like a PROBIOTIC. All in a Fruit! FERMENTED Foods as the ANCIENTS knew (and later worked out by ELIE METCHNIKOFF) confer IMMUNITY to the HOST eater (you). Furthermore, SOUR/SWEET FRUITS keep the GLUCOSE levels down and this helps the body stay away from using its PANCREAS so much—and thereby using INSULIN (which helps speed up AGING). Other pure SWEET FRUITS such as BANANAS or PINEAPPLE have to be eaten sparingly.

REVOLUTIONARY HEALTH INSITE #189: **EAT anything SWEET with something SOUR whenever you do eat FOODS.** Thus, if you eat SWEET POTATOES, you want to make sure to have a glass of WATER with LEMON JUICE squeezed into it as a chaser. PINEAPPLES should be likewise eaten with LEMON JUICE squeezed into the mix. This delays the GLUCOSE hit to the BLOODSTREAM.

REVOLUTIONARY HEALTH INSITE #190: **In General: you need a minimum of 12-16 hours between your LAST meal of the evening and your NEXT meal after waking up from sleep in the morning. This puts the body more in its riteful, Physiological state of KETOSIS *(see Insite #5).*** *Preferably, 20-24 hours would be even better (even 48-96 hours is a great goal to work up to....however, never under other than CRITICAL circumstances go past 6 days of fasting).* Ideally, the first thing in your BODY should be HOT WATER! Then, NO meal until at least 2-4 hours later. If anything must be eaten—it should be SWEET/SOUR FRUIT (ala APPLE, ORANGE, KIWI, PLUMS, LEMONS, LIMES, POMEGRANATE).

We eat too often which causes FOOD PARTICLES to back up in our BLOODSTREAMS which produces MOLD (due to SEPSIS, leading to KANCER, ALLERGIES and so on....this is DISEASE because the body is overworked trying to PROCESS/DIGEST too much food that we have eaten that is now floating around as UNDIGESTED FOOD PARTICLES)! This is made worse, when the Food is a Khemical such as SUGAR which does not digest properly. BACTERIA set up off of this and POISONS our Body. Then, we get things like YEAST, CANDIDA, HEADACHES, TOXEMIA and so on. Or if its WHITE FLOUR we have eaten, the resultant health issue can be ARTHRITIS. This is why we must eat CLEAN as possible–and give our Bodies time to properly Digest the foods we have eaten. You want HOURS of time in between. Additionally, this allows your body to SWITCH over from using its SYMPATHETIC NERVOUS SYSTEM (Digest) to using its PARASYMPATHETIC NERVOUS SYSTEM (Rest and Sleep). Many of us eat too much SUGAR close to our BED TIMES and therefore can not SLEEP well at all! NO SUGAR should be consumed within at least 4 hours of going to BED (if so, it must be done with a BUFFER such as OIL or be combined in a SWEET/SOUR fruit).

REVOLUTIONARY HEALTH INSITE #191: **Children are not meant to be VEGANS! Having your child be a Vegan (when its NOT meant to be one just because you are one) is one of the WORST things you can do!** The child is born out of FAT and continues to need Fat all the way thru the first year. After the FIRST YEAR or TWO a child needs to get its fats from SOLIDS or ANIMAL MEAT (Beef, Bison, Goat, Fish).

REVOLUTIONARY HEALTH INSITE #192: **HUMAN BEINGs must likewise set up their bodies for HIBERNATION (and IMMUNITY) like other Biological Animals with the change of FOODS and the SEAONS.** More foods with a Higher FAT content must be eaten during the FALL/WINTER than SPRING/SUMMER. More ANIMAL SATURATED fat must be eaten during the FALL/WINTER than SPRING/SUMMER (which is the one time when HIGHER levels of CARBOHYDRATES should be eaten to compensate for the ENERGY of the SUNs longer days). For example: Rather than MEAT being 10-20% of your EATIQUETTE (diet) as in the Summer; the ration needs to increase to 30-40% MEAT in the Winter. This is HUMAN HIBERNATION. Lack of ADEQUATE Fat in the Winter is one of the reasons for Increased COLDS, FLUS, PNEUMONIAS, SICKNESS during the Cold Season. Plus, in terms of our VASCULAR SYSTEM, the risk of STROKE is increased in the Winter time because the body takes WATER out of itself; and increases its CLOTTING FACTOR (Fibrinogen)—as a protection against COLD WEATHER (same reason you Winterize your car and put in ANTI-FREEZE). Well, heavier OILS helps prevent this. This especially, helps BLACK people who are not ETHNICALLY from COLD WEATHER. Likewise, please remember that in addition to DARK GREENS and VITAMIN C FRUITS--FATTY MEAT is also an IMMUNE BOOSTER! The KEY? Do Not GORGE yourself on Meat. A few ounces per 10-12 days. We must understand that when the SEASON changes it SHIFTS our body to more reliance on Antioxidant Protective SATURATED FATS, URIC ACID & CARNOSINE which are better ASSIMILATED from MEAT (or MEAT-BY PRODUCTS, ie., EGGS, BUTTER). *(See Insite #141).*

REVOLUTIONARY HEALTH INSITE #193: **CHOLESTEROL will and can INCREASE under STRESS. Therefore, its not unusual to have a HIGH level of Cholesterol if you are in a hectic lifestyle.** In other words, its LESS to do with eating UNHEALTHY (although that can contribute). Rather its often just as much to do with the body PROTECTING your VEINS (VASCULAR SYSTEM) from PRESSURE of your LIFESTYLE. So to say you need to LESSEN your CHOLESTEROL—and give you a STATIN DRUG, for instance--can ENDANGER your health!

REVOLUTIONARY HEALTH INSITE #194: **VITAMIN D is CALCIUM (and CALCIUM is VITAMIN C; its name is dependent on where it is in your body**: ie., in the GUMS/SKIN its VITAMIN C and without it you get SCURVY; however, in the BONES its called CALCIUM....After all, CALCIUM is a SALT—and thatz just what ASCORBIC ACID is too—a SALT! The same SALT. In different parts of the body.; yet it is one and the SAME...however to further confuse the issue: its not CALCIUM we need to be calling it in the bones—rather VITAMIN D is what it really is)!! Thus, you do not need CALCIUM per se, you need VITAMIN D (also a HORMONE/STEROID). From where? The SUN! You ever noticed how hard it is to get VITAMIN D from a FOOD? Your best bet is the SUN (forget about PASTEURIZED MILK...on the other hand, RAW MILK or RAW CHEESE are both good; so is BONE BROTH). Vitamin D is truly a SUNSHINE VITAMIN. Likewise, VITAMIN C has to come from the SUN too (indirectly, however) thru FRUIT....SUN-KISSED fruits! (oranges, apples, berries, strawberries and others). In fact, SUN FOODS are what you want in general. Either DIRECTLY from the SUN or the SUN FOOD itself. This is why its important to EAT more SATURATED FATS/OILS in the Winter: they hold the energy of the SUN the body has collected during the SUMMER! This keeps you from being DEPRESSED; and from losing too much SEROTONIN (a chemical/hormone in the BRAIN that helps you maintain a positive outlook). So it is SCAM to sell you a VITAMIN for VITE D. The body can not process this SYNTHETIC DRUG. Furthermore, the body makes CHOLESTEROL which is turned into VITAMIN D. Therefore, you can never be DEFICIENT in Vitamin D!! (taking drugs or having an unhealthy lifestyle this can mess with your LIVER and this in turn will keep you from Producing CHOLESTEROL which will keep you in turn from making VITAMIN D in the SKIN from the SUN)!! Otherwise, NO PROBLEM with VITAMIN D. And anybody that tells you that is SELLING YOU ON A SCAM—and simply trying to Sell you a PRODUCT!!

REVOLUTIONARY HEALTH INSITE #195: **BOILED WATER is just as effective as DISTILLED WATER—and it is like Drinking the SUN)!** Treat it afterwards with SEA SALT or APPLE CIDER VINEGAR (ACV). Time was you had to go to the CREEK and tote the water back home; now we are going to the GROCERY STORE (and PAYING for the water) and bringing it back home! They still BOIL water in many INDIGENOUS countries and it works for them. Likewise, they give DISTILLED WATER to BABIES in hospitals and its good for them. So DISTILLED or BOILED water is good enough for ANY human to drink as well.

REVOLUTIONARY HEALTH INSITE #196: **According to what I call the C.R.A.C.K (Carbohydrate Restriction And Caloric Ketosis) Diet--the amount of CARBOHYDRATES you EAT should be ONE-FOURTH of your WEIGHT in Ounces of Carbohydrates. Ex: 200 pounds=50 grams of Carbs.** And so on. This keeps us from CONSUMING too many Carbohydrates which break down into GLUCOSE *(which is HARDER on the PANCREAS/body proper than FAT as an ENERGY Source....see Insite #22).* In the same way we use the RULE OF THUMB for Drinking WATER this is how this works, example: HALF your weight in OUNCES of Water is the least amount of water you should drink(200 pounds = 100 ounces of Water).

REVOLUTIONARY HEALTH INSITE #197: **Just as much as the QUALITY of FOOD that you eat—your HEALTH and IMMUNITY is determined just as much by You NOT eating at all!!** In other words, your FASTING (Undereating too) may be the BIGGEST determining FACTOR in your LIFESPAN! Why? Because Eating uses up energy and produces CELL DAMAGE (of course, less so when the quality of your food is more that of WHOLE, LIVE foods that cause relatively little CELL DAMAGE), whereas NOT eating causes NO DAMAGE. Its that simple. In fact, FASTING actually REGENERATES all of the CELLS & TISSUES—as they get a chance to rest. Additionally, mild EXERCISE while FASTING works even Better to RESTORE the body to Increasing YOUTHGEVITY and spurring on LONGEVITY! An ideal fast is 24-96 hours on WATER and/or JUICES, alternating (if you can stand it otherwise 48 hours is great). Do this every 12 days. This addresses both CALORIC and CARBOHYDRATE RESTRICTION together.

REVOLUTIONARY HEALTH INSITE #198: **The ability of the body to Increase the Hormone MOTILIN (when NOT eating) and reduce the Hormone GHRELIN in the STOMACH is what turns on our LONGEVITY GENES (SIRT GENES they call them).** The same ones that the Chemical RESVERATROL is allegedly switching on, enabling ANIMALS to live longer. GHRELIN signals HUNGER. Whereas MOTILIN suppresses HUNGER Signals. Yet, its NOT detrimental and you lose no HEALTH because at the same time the HYPOTHALAMUS signals the body to Release its FAT stores and this gives you the feeling of SAIETY (fullness)—NO HUNGER! Living this way allows you to SURVIVE and THRIVE and avoid the INSULIN SWINGS of HUNGER (GHRELIN). This is what HELPS you. When you look at the history of our Ancestors, the fact that they were often not able to eat worked in their favor—enabling their DIGESTIVE SYSTEMS to take a rest—and as a result INCREASING their lifespans (they lived much longer than we do today because they were not ALWAYS eating; whether this was on Purpose or simply due to not having enuff food—however, it worked. And rite today CALORIC RESTRICTION is the #1 reason that all ANIMALS that have been studied have doubled their LIFESPANS). This was due to MOTILIN (and FAT/GLUCAGON) rather than GHRELIN (and SUGAR/GLUCOSE) playing more of a role in the EATING CYCLE! You can induce MOTILIN thru FASTING, UNDEREATING, WATER DRINKING and EXERCISE. Thus, all the rage about RESVERATROL owes its hype to the Mechanism of MOTILIN, actually. It works hand in hand with those aforementioned SIRTUIN GENES to increase LIFESPANS.

REVOLUTIONARY HEALTH INSITE #199: **We are facing an EPIDEMIC of the LACK of the really SMALL Nutrient: the NANO NUTRIENTS (BORON, CESIUM, RUBIDIUM, STRONTIUM).** These Nutrients are even smaller than MICRONUTRIENTS. And we barely realize they are there in the BODY Proper until its nearly TOO LATE! These NANO NUTRIENTS will be behind much of the DIS-EASE we will be facing going forwards. BORON is needed to Hold the VITAMIN D in the BONES; CESIUM is needed to balance the PH of your CELLS).

REVOLUTIONARY HEALTH INSITE #200: **The CURE for AGING is to ELIMINATE....All....SUGAR (so that you SPARE your PANCREAS**....*see Insite #22)!!* Repeat: STOP....ALL....SUGAR. CONSUMPTION! The PSEUDO-SCIENTISTS and the FRANKENMEDS keep telling us about all the CAUSES for AGING including INFLAMMATION, FREE RADICAL CELL DAMAGE, INFECTION, VIRUS, BACTERIA, MOLD and GENETICS. Yet, as IMPORTANT as these are in the EQUATION of Aging—they are essentially

SYMPTOMS

of Aging and NOT the

CAUSE

of AGING! They do contribute to Aging. But the real cause for AGING is

SUGAR!

C12 H22 O11 (the chemical symbol for Sugar)....

....or said another way: too much Damn SYNTHETIC GLUCOSE in your BLOODSTREAM!! Sugar in all its SYNTHETIC, PROCESSED, REFINED, RECONSTITUTED—Forms......in DRINKS, SODAS, JUICES, BREADS, PASTAS, CANNED FOODS, COOKIES, SNACKS, POTATO CHIPS, CANDY, PACKAGED GOODS—all are FULL of Sugar. And housing a DANGERSOUS, KILLING, AGING Substance. Khemical. Additive. Poison. Toxemia. One which steady promotes every DISEASE known to HUMANITY: including AUTOIMMUNE, DIABETES, WRINKLES, OSTEOPOROSIS, SENILE DEMENTIA, PARKINSONS, ALZHEIMERS, MULTIPLE SCLEROSIS,

SCHIZOPHRENIA, AIDS, CANCER............Putting Sugar in your body is no different than putting Sugar in the TANK of your Car! Your body does not need to run off of Sugar. It needs to run PRIMARILY off of

FAT!

Otherwise Sugar does not need to enter the body other than as part of the Normal BREAKDOWN of eating LIVE, WHOLE, DENSE foods! Because this is how your body is supposed to obtain its GLUCOSE. Natural GLUCOSE. Not the Synthetic CRAP that comes from Refined Carbohydrates and Processed Foods and other Packaged junk foods. Your body can not breakdown Synthetic Sugar. And it BUILDS UP in the BLOODSTREAM giving you what the old folks call "that Sugar." Your body uses/needs NATURAL Sugar. All kinds of other Sugar SPOILS, ROTTENS your CELLS from the inside-out. It SMOTHERS them, resulting in the CELLS being prohibited from getting what Dr. OTTO WARBURG called CELL RESPIRATION. Lack of OXYGEN. Functioning at in ANAEROBIC CAPACITY rather than an AEROBIC one. Due to Sugar that has FERMENTED in/around those Cells. Where there is NO OXYGEN there is NO LIFE! This further creates a GAS much like a MUSTARD GAS during War time which stops the Cells ability to BREATHE (just like a Human being who was breathing GAS). Any type of Food that is SYNTHETIC, FAKE, PROCESSED, REFINED like HEATED OILS, FRIED MEATS, ADDITIVES, DYES, PRESERVATIVES, SMOKE, POLLUTION—will stop the RESPIRATION of your Cells---this is KANCER, ALLERGIES and other kinds of DISEASES. So if you want to stop AGING------then STOP the Ingestion of SUGAR and other chemicals. Especially, Sugar which turn out to be POISON to the CELLULAR STRUCTURE. You can EAT whatever you want provided it is LIVE, WHOLE, NUTRIENT & PROTEIN DENSE. A Real Source food. This is how you cure Aging. No FAKE FOODS. Foods that have been made in a Laboratory and put into a

PACKAGE, CRATE, and so on complete with ADDITIVES and PRESERVATIVES added to it!! Meanwhile, SUGAR is the LOWEST form of energy known to man that we have been convinced that we must EAT to operate our Bodies. DEAD Sugar. Rather than LIVE FAT! SOUR/SWEET SUGARS. Yes, not this crude COCAINEnish Sugar! If you leave Sugar alone you will not only CURE Aging—you will REVERSE Aging! You will SLOW DOWN Aging to a crawl! You will rarely be SICK again.

Very key in cases of DETOXIFICATION, especially, if you are trying to Stop SMOKING, DRUGS and so on.

The 6-Day Six-Cess Detox System

Day 1 – 24 hrs of drinking only distilled water*

Day 2 – Eat only fruits

Day 3 – 24 hrs of drinking only fruit juices

Day 4 - Eat only vegetables and salads

Day 5 – 24 hrs of drinking only vegetable juices

Day 6 – Eat fruit & vegetable salad combined on separately

Day 7 – Ease back into your normal diet with a lite meal

*hypoglycemics should eat fruit on Day 1

The LACK OF CEREMONY

We do not have CEREMONY in our lives anymore. The LACK of a SACRED RITUAL or RITE OF PASSAGE has caused us to become de-linked from a life of meaning. And from one another.

If we are to be RE-CONNECTED TO ONE ANOTHER WE must have a RITUAL that HEALS us as a family unit, even as it brings us together. For it is this LACK which keeps many of us as a People in a STATE OF POST TRAUMATIC STRESS/SLAVE DISORDER. Additionally, it is causing many of our CHILDREN to be LEFT BEHIND with no direction for their lives. How can our CHILDREN have DIRECTION if they have no CONNECTION? The RITE of PASSAGE GIVES THEM THIS, however.

Since many of our YOUNG ones can not find or get this CONNECTION from their Biological family, they SEEK it elsewhere, and often in places that are ultimately, not spiritually beneficial – GANGS for example or DRUGS. And simply just the STREETS!

Perhaps, if we understood the PROCESS of becoming a MAN or WOMAN, WE WOULD BE ABLE TO SEE THE BEST path in which to DIRECT OUR BELOVED children, even OURSEELVES! Every ANCIENT culture that truly CARED about their young embraced the RITE OF PASSAGE. You see, for the CHILD will go through the process WITH or WITHOUT your help. In other words, with RITE KNOWLEDGE or without RITE KNOWLEDGE – and this makes the difference in whether or not the CHILD goes on to become a PRODUCTIVE or UNPRODCTIVE part of the FAMILY, COMMUNITY, SOCIETY unit!

There are 6 important steps and they are listed below:

SEPARATION

ISOLATION

MEDITATION

EDUCATION

REINCORPORATION

APPLICATION

By Dr. Moo-Twahz

www.thepeopleshealer.com

INDEX

T

U

V

W

Z

LaVergne, TN USA
13 January 2010
169860LV00005B/1/P

9 780984 393701